Statistics in Public Health

Statistics in Public Health
Qualitative Approaches to Public Health Problems

Donna F. Stroup, Ph.D., M.Sc.
Steven M. Teutsch, M.D., M.P.H.

New York   Oxford
Oxford University Press
1998

Oxford University Press

Oxford   New York
Athens   Auckland   Bangkok   Bogota
Bombay   Buenos Aires   Calcutta   Cape Town
Dar es Salaam   Delhi   Florence   Hong Kong   Istanbul
Karachi   Kuala Lumpur   Madras   Madrid
Melbourne   Mexico City   Nairobi   Paris
Singapore   Taipei   Tokyo   Toronto   Warsaw

and associated companies in
Berlin   Ibadan

Published by Oxford University Press, Inc.
198 Madison Avenue, New York, New York 10016

Oxford is a registered trademark of Oxford University Press

Library of Congress Cataloging-in-Publication Data
Stroup, Donna F.
    Statistics in public health : quantitative approaches to public
health problems / Donna F. Stroup, Steven M. Teutsch.
        p.   cm.   Includes bibliographical references and index.
ISBN 0–19–511498–1
    1. Public health surveillance—Pennsylvania.
    2. Health risk assessment—Statistical methods.
I. Teutsch, Steven M.   II. Title.
    RA652.2.P82S77   1988   614.4'07'27—DC21
    DNLM/DLC   for Library of Congress   97-47073
                                                         Rev.

1   3   5   7   9   8   6   4   2

Printed in the United States of America
on acid-free paper

Foreword

The health of the people is the bedrock on which our social progress is built. There is a continuing need for accurately measuring and monitoring changes and improvements in the health of populations by preventing and reducing environmental and occupational hazards and promoting health, enhancing personal behavior, as well as improving the effectiveness of our health care system. Public health encompasses many and varying complex activities for preventing disease and promoting health, including immunizations, identification and control of epidemics and potential hazards in the environment, injury prevention, and the promotion of better health habits. Because of the increasing complexities of public health problems and activities, we need to bring to bear a wide array of quantitative approaches and solutions to these problems. This book provides an important guide and resource that relates statistical methods to core public health functions that form the scientific basis for policy development, priority setting, and management in public health.

The health of populations is largely determined by their social, economic, and physical environment, as well as health behaviors and medical care. Public health policy requires multidisciplinary, multifaceted, and multisectorial approaches to promoting health and preventing disease. Health policy makers, decision makers, researchers, and managers have a compelling need for better data and appropriate analytical tools to assess existing health care policies and to anticipate the need for, and consequences of, policy changes. This book will help these persons by providing an excellent and comprehensive overview of statistical and other quantitative methods required to better assess these public health functions and to guide the reader in the application of these methods to public health.

The book is written with the basic understanding that public health relies upon quantitative methods and the long history of science serving policy development, priority setting, and management. This book first presents a historical perspective on quantitative methods in public health, followed by a review of the basic concepts of statistics important in solving practical public health problems and appropriate use. Included are probability theory, statistical inference, measurement of risk, sampling, significance testing and confidence interval estimation, modeling, logistic regression, mutivariable analysis, attributable risk, and forecasting. The wide range of data sources for public health at the local, state, and national levels are reviewed.

The remainder of the book deals with practical applications in public health: health monitoring and strategies for identifying and collecting the information necessary to attain disease prevention and health promotion goals, investigating health effects and hazard in the community, quantitative tools available to help public health decision makers understand the effectiveness and value of options available to them, statistical techniques used in developing public health guidelines and policies, conceptual and statistical issues for implementing and monitoring programs, and methodologies involved in design of effective program evaluation.

As a health services researcher and former Director of the National Center for Health Statistics, the part of the Centers for Disease Control and Prevention (CDC) responsible by law for the collection, analysis, and dissemination of statistics on the health of the nation, I am acutely aware that statisticians, health services researchers, epidemiologists, social scientists, and others are increasingly expected to provide the keys to national decision-making in the health field. This encompasses many global problems, including uneven quality of and access to medical care, increasing strain on available resources, persistently rising medical care costs, environmental pollution, poor nutrition, and poor health behaviors. Knowledge of and competence in the application of statistical principles and techniques are required for understanding, analyzing, and finding practical solutions to these problems. I welcome this book and its contributions to the advancement of quantitative solutions to public health problems.

Dorothy P. Rice

Preface

Public health deals with the prevention of disease, disability, and death in human populations. Just as clinical medicine has the individual as its unit of study, public health science and practice have the aggregate population as the unit of analysis. Thus, statistical methods that deal with aggregates of measurements provide the scientific basis for identifying health problems, establishing objectives for health promotion and for disease and injury prevention, setting priorities for the allocation of health care resources, and determining the impact of specific interventions. Other quantitative methods, such as economics, decision theory, and deterministic mathematics, now form integral parts of the scientific basis of priority setting and evaluation in public health.

Before 1850, the word *statistics* was used in a different sense than the present one. It literally meant "information about the state." Public health still acknowledges this usage, since "vital statistics," information on births and deaths in the nation, is one of the oldest and most widely used data systems for public health. In addition, methods of statistical analysis are integral to the practice of public health in every area. Forecasting influenza seasons, measuring the effect of lead in gasoline, quantifying the burden of disease, detecting emergent problems in human populations, setting priorities for health services to be covered in managed care, measuring the effectiveness of prevention activities: these are but a few areas where statistics contributes to the health of the population.

Although numerous texts cover the theory and methods of epidemiology and biostatistics, no single resource has been available to guide analysts in the application of these methods in public health. This book is intended to be used as a desk reference for those practicing public health and as a textbook for students in degree programs in public health. It gives broad conceptual treatment to the statistical issues underlying basic public health functions and provides a reference to sources for more complete technical explanations. The individual chapters integrate theory and application to provide a concise overview relating statistical methods to core public health functions. The book will serve as a companion to other Oxford texts from CDC such as *Principles and Practice of Public Health*

Surveillance; Prevention Effectiveness: A Guide to Decision Analysis and Economic Evaluation; and *Field Epidemiology.*

We have divided the book into two sections. Chapters 1–3 deal with the history and fundamentals of quantitative methods in public health: basic concepts of statistics, public health surveillance, public health surveys, public health information systems, and the communication of information to form and carry out public health policy. Chapters 4–8 adopt the framework of core public health functions (The Ten Organizational Practices of Public Health, Am J Prev Med 1995; 11 (Suppl 6) 6–8): outbreak investigations, policy development, economic and program evaluation, managed care, and program operations. Although most examples are drawn from public health activities in the United States, they illustrate methodologies that can be applied in many other parts of the world.

We would like to acknowledge the contributions of Dr. Manning Feinleib, who commented on the outline and early drafts of the manuscript; Ms. Barbara P. McDonnell, who expertly managed a complex array of information for numerous chapter drafts; and Ms. Rachel Wilson, who edited early drafts.

Atlanta, Ga.   D. F. S.
West Point, Pa.   S. M. T.

Contents

Contributors

JOHN S. ANDREWS, JR., M.D., M.P.H.
Associate Administrator for Science
Agency for Toxic Substances and
  Disease Registry
Atlanta, Georgia

NANCY D. BARKER, M.S.
Statistician
Atlanta, Georgia

RUTH L. BERKELMAN, M.D.
Senior Advisor to Director, CDC
Centers for Disease Control and
  Prevention
Atlanta, Georgia

ROSS C. BROWNSON, Ph.D.
Professor and Chair
Department of Community Health
  and Prevention Research Center
School of Public Health
St. Louis University
St. Louis, Missouri

OWEN DEVINE, Ph.D.
Statistician
Radiation Studies Branch
National Center for Environmental
  Health
Centers for Disease Control and
  Prevention
Atlanta Georgia

MICHAEL HENNESSY, Ph.D., MPH
Behavioral Scientist
Behavioral Interventions and Research
  Branch
Division of Sexually Transmitted
  Disease Prevention
Centers for Disease Control and
  Prevention
Atlanta, Georgia

ALAN R. HINMAN, M.D., M.P.H.
Senior Consultant for Public Health
  Programs
The Task Force for Child Survival &
  Development
Atlanta, Georgia

KAREN KAFADAR, Ph.D.
Professor
Department of Mathematics
University of Colorado at Denver
Denver, Colorado

MARTIN MELTZER, B.Sc. Agric. (Hons),
  MS., Ph.D.
Economist and Senior Staff Fellow
Office of the Director
National Center for Infectious Diseases
Centers for Disease Control and
  Prevention
Atlanta, Georgia

R. GIBSON PARRISH, M.D.
Senior Epidemiologist
Surveillance and Programs Branch
National Center for Environmental
    Health
Centers for Disease Control and
    Prevention
Atlanta, Georgia

EDUARDO J. SIMOES, M.D., M.Sc., M.P.H.
Chronic Disease Epidemiologist
Division of Chronic Disease
    Prevention and Health Promotion
Missouri Department of Health
St. Louis, Missouri

DIXIE E. SNIDER, JR., M.D., M.P.H.
Associate Director for Science
Centers for Disease Control and
    Prevention
Atlanta, Georgia

DONNA F. STROUP, Ph.D., M.Sc.
Associate Director for Science
Epidemiology Program Office
Centers for Disease Control and
    Prevention
Atlanta, Georgia

STEVEN M. TEUTSCH, M.D., M.P.H.
Senior Research Scientist
Outcomes Research & Management
Merck & Co., Inc.
West Point, Pennsylvania
Formerly Director, Division of
    Prevention Research and Analytic
    Methods
Epidemiology Program Office
Centers for Disease Control and
    Prevention
Atlanta, Georgia

STEPHEN B. THACKER, M.D., M.Sc.
Director
Epidemiology Program Office
Centers for Disease Control and
    Prevention
Atlanta, Georgia

SCOTT F. WETTERHALL, M.D., M.P.H.
Medical Epidemiologist
Office of Program Planning and
    Evaluation
Centers for Disease Control and
    Prevention
Atlanta, Georgia

ELIZABETH R. ZELL, MS
Data Management Branch
Biomedical Statistician
National Immunization
    Program
Centers for Disease Control and
    Prevention
Atlanta, Georgia

Statistics in Public Health

1

History of Statistical Methods in Public Health

DONNA F. STROUP
RUTH L. BERKELMAN

> Science and technology revolutionize our lives, but memory, tradition, and myth frame our response.
>
> —Arthur M. Schlesinger, Jr. (1917–)

While clinical medicine has the individual as its focus, *public health* is fundamentally concerned with preventing disease, disability, and premature death in the population or community. Because of this focus on populations rather than individuals, statistics and other numerical methods that deal with aggregates of measurements provide the scientific basis for basic public health tasks: identifying public health problems, establishing objectives for health promotion and disease and injury prevention, setting priorities for the allocation of health care resources, and determining the impact of specific interventions. *Statistics,* the science of finding underlying patterns by analyzing variability and errors in observed data (Rose, 1985; Murray, 1993), is essential to understanding problems of disease in human populations because of widespread variation in social systems and biology (Sladen and Bang, 1969).

The history of the use of statistics in epidemiology and public health frames its relevance to current problems. In a recent history of Europe, the author comments on the scope of any historical endeavor: "History can be written at any magnification. One can write the history of the universe on a single page, or the life-cycle of a mayfly in forty volumes" (Davies, 1996). This chapter will not provide a comprehensive account of the origins of every method; rather, its purpose is to explore important events in the development of statistics in public health. We will describe the roots of many common statistical concepts that are applied to public health, with emphasis on methods used to establish policy.

Statistics and Public Health Policy

"The basic operation of the epidemiologist is to count cases and measure the population in which they arise" (Langmuir, 1987). With this statement, Alexander D. Langmuir articulated the critical role of statistical methods in public health practice. The collaboration between statisticians and epidemiologists has led to advances in both disciplines (Ethridge, 1992; Fee, 1987). Statisticians have developed methods that epidemiologists have adopted as their own (Greenberg and Kleinbaum, 1985; Kahn and Sempos, 1989), and epidemiologists have posed questions that have led to the development of new statistical methods (Robins and Greenland, 1986; Stroup et al., 1989; Thompson, 1991). On the other hand, this alliance of fields has sometimes generated controversy (Charlton, 1996; Taubes, 1995; Davidson, 1994) over the application of quantitative information to human populations.

The collaboration between statistics and epidemiology in public health practice leads to the practice of *consequential statistics*—the application of statistical methods to important problems affecting human communities (e.g., acquired immunodeficiency syndrome [AIDS], influenza, suicide, and immunization). Because of the importance of these issues in the health of our communities, the results of this statistical science must withstand the scrutiny not only of peer reviewers for scientific journals but also of local newspapers, politicians, and public advocacy groups (Shy, 1997). Geoffrey Watson described the consequential context of statistics as follows (D. F. Stroup, personal communication, 1975):

> "Small-scale" science, where experiments can be planned to investigate a particular point is what much of theoretical statistics has in mind. In environmental work or in mandating the use of helmets for cyclists, things are very different. One has to make do with what is available and seems relevant, whether it is truly representative or not. Instruments may vary from place to place, outliers are very common. . . . The trade of a statistician is consequential, not confined to what we teach or read in statistical textbooks.

An example can be found in the controversy arising from the projection of AIDS incidence in the United States. The *normal (gaussian) distribution* is a fundamental mathematical form used to model the occurrence of a wide range of natural phenomena (Kendall and Stuart, 1969). Sometimes, when data are not normally distributed, a mathematical transformation can be used to more closely achieve a normal distribution; for example, the natural logarithm of each data value may more closely approximate the normal distribution than do the raw data themselves (Velleman and Hoaglin, 1981). This process produces a *lognormal distribution,* which has been used to model the intensity of incidence during influenza epidemics (Sartwell, 1950). In the early years of the AIDS epidemic, Langmuir and his statistical colleague Dennis Bregman used this lognormal model to predict total incidence of AIDS cases in the United States (Bregman and Langmuir, 1990; Artzrouni, 1990). Subsequent data collection showed that the lognormal model substantially underpredicted the actual course of the epidemic (Gail and Brookmeyer, 1990). The failure of the model to predict the actual course of the epidemic was due to the unapparent presence of multiple heterogeneous risk groups (e.g., homosexuals, heterosexuals, intravenous drug users), rather than any underlying flaw in statistical methodology. The examples of effectiveness of folic acid in preventing neural tube defects and the effectiveness of mammography screening among women aged 40–49 in reducing mortality from breast cancer (Canadian Task Force on the Periodic Health Examination, 1994) provide further evidence that the scrutiny of statistical methods in epidemiology is not unique.

Vital Statistics

Statistics and human lives have been linked since early tribal societies used data from artifacts and skeletons to make inferences about their populations (Lancaster, 1990), although the terminology has evolved. As early as the Italian Renaissance, information about the health of a city's population became widely available (Rosen, 1958). The first recorded use of the term *biometry* was by William Whewell in 1831 in reference to "calculations on lives" (Burchfield, 1972). Before 1850, the word *statistics* literally meant "information about the state." This meaning still survives, in that "vital statistics"—data on births and deaths—refers to one of the oldest and most widely used data systems for public health (Lambert, 1963) (see Chapter 3).

The term "political arithmetic" was coined by Sir William Petty, who used mathematical methods to study mortality among hospital patients (Rosen, 1958). In 1665, Petty's friend, John Graunt, authored the classic book *Observations upon Bills of Mortality;* which provides the earliest example of the use of statistics to monitor the health of a population. Graunt showed for the first time a differential in health status and mortality between urban and rural populations (Greenwood, 1948). Perhaps Graunt's greatest contribution to statistics in public health was to recognize that the usefulness of mathematical analyses is limited by the quality of the original data.

Graunt's efforts influenced Christian Huygens, who, in 1693, mathematically determined the expectation of life at any age (Rosen, 1958). This *life-table* approach was used by the first insurance companies that were established in London. The development of life-table methodology and subsequent survival analytic approaches has spanned almost 350 years (Lancaster, 1990) and is still an active area of research (Dwyer and Feinleib, 1988).

Later, William Farr (1807–83), a physician with a love for statistics, was the first to use vital records quantitatively to study epidemics:

> Medical science will advance not by vague speculations, opinions and assertions but by registering facts, employing the microscope, by chemical analysis, weighing and measuring phenomena, determining their relations and by applying that mighty instrument of natural science—arithmetic and mathematics. (Farr, 1837)

Using such techniques from mathematics, Farr demonstrated statistically the correlation between mortality from cholera and pollution of water supplies; similarly, he was able to document the reduction in mortality attributable to English sanitary measures. Farr developed an early application of forecasting methodology to show both the disastrous effect of continued illiteracy (Greenwood, 1948) and the economic consequences of disease (Langmuir, 1976). In a biography of pioneers of social medicine, Greenwood wrote:

> It has been said that a vital statistician spends his life on the records of human sorrow, deaths and more deaths, nice, neat records, tidy columns of figures with all the tears wiped off. Some vital statisticians saw the tears; Farr did. (Greenwood, 1948)

Greenwood's words are echoed in 1983 by Secretary of State Henry Kissinger in conversation with William Foege, the son of a Lutheran missionary and former director of the Centers for Disease Control and Prevention (CDC), about the number of persons starving in Nigeria: "For me, those are numbers; for you, they must be faces" (Ethridge, 1992).

Farr's teachings were broadly influential. In the mid-1800s, John Simon entered public service in Britain and used a combination of morbidity data and data from sanitation engineering assessment to address the problem of malaria (Simon, 1890). Another student of Farr, Florence Nightingale, presented a paper to the International Statistical Conference in London in 1860 in which she related total mortality data to the number of hospital beds available. Although such a simple index may be misleading (e.g., a function of the fatality of the disease and the duration of treatment), Nightingale argued forcefully for statistical education "in order to legislate for and to administer our national life with more precision and experience" (Greenwood, 1948).

Beginning in the early 1900s, registration of vital events in the United States was complete enough to be useful in periods not covered by the decennial census (Rice, 1981). For most of the twentieth century, birth and death registration were separate systems; in 1988, however, the National Center for Health Statistics linked files of death certificates of infants dying before 1 year of age to their birth certificates, thereby providing valuable information (e.g., prenatal care) for causes of infant death (Feinleib, 1995). On the other hand, the International Classification of Diseases (ICD) codes used for categorizing causes of death in vital records are based on organ systems, which may be less useful for public health because they may not point to specific causes or prevention activities (Irvine et al., 1984). Vital statistics systems in the twenty-first century will meet new challenges of automated reporting of births and deaths (Hanzlick, 1994; Israel, 1990) and improvements in the reporting of race and ethnicity (Farley et al., 1995; Hahn and Eberhardt, 1990).

Public Health Surveillance

In addition to data on vital statistics, other aspects of populations have been monitored in public health practice. *Public health surveillance* is the ongoing and systematic collection, analysis, and interpretation of outcome-specific health data, closely integrated with the timely dissemination of these data to those responsible for preventing and controlling disease or injury (see Chapter 3). The link between public health surveillance and statistics is illustrated by Lemuel Shattuck, who both outlined the basis for a public health organization that included data collection for surveillance (Shattuck, 1848) and helped to establish the American Statistical Association. The history of public health surveillance can be traced back to efforts to control the bubonic plague in the fourteenth century (Thacker, 1992). The first use of scientifically based surveillance concepts in public health practice was the monitoring of contacts of persons who had serious communicable diseases (e.g., plague, smallpox, typhus, and yellow fever) to detect the first signs and symptoms of disease and to begin prompt isolation. The association between the arrival of ships and spread of disease, first observed with surveillance during the polio pandemic of 1917–18 (Ohadike, 1991), gave impetus to monitoring by foreign quarantine stations throughout the world.

In the late 1940s, Alexander D. Langmuir, then the chief epidemiologist of the Communicable Disease Center (now the Centers for Disease Control and Prevention), began to broaden this concept of surveillance (Thacker and Gregg, 1996). Although surveillance of persons at risk for specific diseases continued at quarantine stations, Langmuir and his colleagues shifted the focus of surveillance to the occurrence of specific diseases in populations, rather than in individuals. They emphasized the rapid collection and analysis of data on a particular disease and the quick dissemination of the findings to those who could use them for prevention and intervention efforts (Langmuir, 1963). As later stated by Foege et al. (1976): "The reason for collecting, analyzing, and disseminating information on a disease is to control that disease. Collection and analysis should not be allowed to consume resources if action does not follow." Although surveillance activities originally involved protection of the population against infectious diseases (Langmuir, 1963), more recently a variety of health events (e.g., childhood lead poisoning, birth defects, injuries, cancer, diabetes mellitus, and behavioral risk factors) have been included in national and state surveillance activities (Thacker and Stroup, 1994).

Sampling in Medicine/Public Health

Techniques of *sampling* were used in the eighteenth century by James Lind, a physician from Edinburgh, to show (in an early clinical trial) that scurvy, a disease costing thousands of lives annually, could not only be cured but also prevented by consuming fruits containing citric acid (Lind, 1953). In an early application of statistics in public health policy, the British Navy acted on Lind's analysis and required the inclusion of limes or lime juice in the diet on ships (thus, the nickname "limeys" for British seamen).

Later, as the French Revolution stimulated an interest in public health and preventive medicine, Pierre Charles-Alexander Louis used sampling to determine that bloodletting was not an efficacious treatment and reversed a trend of increasing use of this practice by physicians (Louis, 1836). Louis' work had far-reaching implications for the study of typhoid fever (Budd, 1931) and cholera (Snow, 1936). In 1926, R. A. Fisher introduced a term for this sampling process—*randomization,* the use of principles of probability to disperse the sample throughout the population and reduce biases due to confounding (Fisher, 1926).

Several public health efforts illustrate the pivotal role of sampling. In France, population estimates were made by using the number of residents in sampled districts, the number of births and deaths in those samples, and the numbers of births and deaths in the entire country. Sir Frederick Morton Eden calculated a population estimate by sampling households from tax rolls (Deming and Stuart, 1968). Surveillance and survey sampling were instrumental in the development of vaccines for polio during the 1950s (Serfling and Sherman, 1965). The sample design of the National Health and Examination Survey played a pivotal role in the elimination of lead from gasoline (Annest et al., 1983), and sampling methodology continues to inform rapid assessments following natural disasters (Centers for Disease Control and Prevention, 1992).

Estimation and Significance Testing

The process of estimation refers to methods of using probability to obtain approximate answers that are likely to be close to exact values, when the latter are not easily obtainable. For example, an early practical application of probability to the measurement of variability was used to account for migration and other factors in obtaining an estimate for a population census (Quetelet, 1827). *Least squares estimation* was developed by choosing an estimator that minimizes the sum of all possible "errors" between the estimator and the actual data (Legendre, 1805; Laplace, 1786). Quetelet adapted the method of least squares estimation to develop an early ratio estimate for the complete census of a country not by enumeration, but by incorporating data from a sample of communities and birth registries (Quetelet, 1828). With this methodology he analyzed the effect of atmospheric temperature on the rates of births and deaths. Further, Quetelet compared rates of alcohol abuse and violent crime to formulate early concepts of causality (Quetelet, 1835; see section Development of Study Designs, later in this chapter) and to interpret probabilities as epidemiological rates of disease (Stigler, 1986). The utility of rates was extended by Siméon Denis Poisson, the discoverer of the mathematical model (statistical distribution) that now bears his name, when he developed methods to quantify the uncertainty associated with small rates.

Development of Study Designs

The application of statistics to public health problems in the nineteenth century was impeded by the heterogeneity of human populations. To apply existing statistical theory, epidemiologists had to assume that variation within groups of people was structurally equivalent to random variations in natural phenomena (e.g., weather) (Stigler, 1986). The heterogeneity of populations (e.g., decisions to vaccinate a child were seldom random, but were perhaps related to other healthy or risky behaviors) led to a two-pronged approach to addressing public health problems: the development of tests of homogeneity (Lexis, 1877) and the development of study designs to control for sources of variation (Pierce and Jastrow, 1885). We briefly review the development of selected examples of study designs in epidemiology and public health.

The *cross-sectional field survey,* observations on variables at a point of time, has advantages over other study designs due to sample availability, independence of observations, and reliability (Mundlak, 1978). This study design was used as early as 1916 to study cotton mill communities at risk for pellagra (Goldberger et al., 1918). Following World War II, this technique was used in national morbidity surveys (The Commission on Chronic Illness, 1956).

The *case-control study* uses a design that compares prior exposures in people who have a particular illness or other health event with people who do not (Kahn and Sempos, 1989). Early case-control studies were first used to investigate rare events, since the design offers sampling efficiency for this situation (Broders, 1920; Lane-Claypon, 1926; Lombard and Doering, 1928; Lilienfeld and Lilienfeld, 1979). Gustav Theodor Fechner used this design to investigate how different factors affected individual judgment (Fechner, 1860). Another early example of the case-control methodology is a 1843 study of pulmonary consumption (Lilienfeld and Lilienfeld, 1979). The case-control study design may be one of the most remarkable contributions of statistics to epidemiology (Gross, 1976; Breslow, 1996). The first systematic discussion of the *cohort study* design appeared in 1960 (MacMahon et al., 1960). In this situation, subsets of the population of interest are identified and followed to ascertain exposure status and subsequent development of disease or injury. Its classical application in epidemiology can be found in the Framingham Study (Dawber, 1980). As a result of support from Dr. Joseph Mountin, Assistant Surgeon General, the study was initiated in 1947 to assess the rising epidemic of heart disease. It provides data to illustrate the distinction between cumulative incidence and period incidence of chronic diseases, variability of repeated measurement over time, and stopping rules for a longitudinal study (Winslow et al., 1952).

Designs such as the cohort study and *cross-sectional community studies,* which examine the relationship between health events and other factors of potential interest as they exist at a single point in time, are often expensive or difficult to conduct. As a result, case-control studies began to dominate American epidemiology more broadly in the 1950s (Cole, 1979). The technique of matching, commonly used to address issues of confounding, was first used for hospital controls in studying breast cancer (Lane-Claypon, 1926). The Broders study of squamous cell epithelioma of the lip showed that although tobacco use was similar in cases and controls, their method of smoking differed markedly—cases were more likely to smoke pipes (Broders, 1920).

Following World War II, epidemiological applications of the case-control study increased (Schreck and Lenowitz, 1947; Sartwell, 1947; Schreck et al., 1950; Wynder and Graham, 1950; Levin et al., 1950). Important contributions to the theory and practice of case-control studies made possible their more widespread application in epidemiology. Examples include Cornfield's demonstration that the odds ratio can be used in both cohort and case-control study designs (Cornfield, 1951), the Mantel-Haenszel estimate and related procedures for dependent (e.g., before-and-after) data (Mantel-Haenszel, 1959), and recent work concerning nested study designs (Breslow, 1996).

Forecasting

The ability to *forecast trends* in data can provide a fundamental aid to public health decisions. Forecasting is generally done either graphically, or analytically using mathematical models. An early example of graphical methods in forecasting can be found in Edward Shakespeare's report on cholera in Europe and India (Shakespeare, 1890). The first documented use of data to construct a mathematical model to forecast trends in public health was by William Farr in his use of vital statistics and a logistic model to show that illiteracy in communities is adversely related to length of life (Farr, 1837; Lancaster, 1990; Greenwood, 1948).

Since that time, forecasting techniques have been used in the surveillance of influenza, with both statistical (Stroup et al., 1988) and deterministic (Thacker and

Stroup, 1990) models. For example, a mathematical model based on *network theory* has been used to model the global effect of influenza using information from the initial city of incidence (Rvachev and Longini, 1985). Network theory uses the direction of movement of systems in channels (e.g., roads or air traffic patterns) to make forecasts or predictions (Haggett et al., 1977). The important use of these forecasting models in elimination campaigns is shown in the work of Dr. George Macdonald that was critical to the successful elimination of measles from The Gambia in 1969 (Thacker and Millar, 1991). Similar methods have been applied to data on sexually transmitted diseases (Schnell et al., 1989; Zaidi et al., 1989).

The statistical issues that arise concerning the statistics of the AIDS epidemic illustrate the impact of statistical forecasting in epidemiology (Brookmeyer, 1996). In this work, the traditional method of extrapolation of curves proved insufficient to forecast cases of AIDS because of reporting delays (Bregman and Langmuir, 1990; Gail and Brookmeyer, 1990) and incompleteness of exposure data (Lui et al., 1986). The *back-calculation method,* which allows the estimation of exposure distributions from reported incidence data (Brookmeyer and Gail, 1986), was developed to address these problems but became less useful with the introduction of retroviral and other therapy that lengthened the incubation period (Brookmeyer, 1996; Houweling and Coutinho, 1997) and with changes in case definition (Buehler et al., 1993). Use of biomarkers and surveys has been proposed as an alternative to the back-calculation method (Brookmeyer and Quinn, 1995).

Multivariable Techniques

The increasing use of the *field survey* following World War II was associated with the health problems created by the conflict. This type of study could not reliably ascertain temporal order and thus posed the risk of creating confounding causal relationships. To address this problem, social scientists began to use multivariable analysis (Fisher, 1925). One multivariable technique, *path analysis,* which creates causal models from postulated relationships, was invented at the time of World War I (Wright, 1978) but was not used in biomedicine until the 1970s. The first specification of a modeling strategy to examine causality can be found in MacMahon et al. (1960). However, widespread use of the method did not occur until the development of *multiple regression* and *logistic regression* (Suits, 1957), since these methods allowed for estimation of coefficients with epidemiologic interpretation.

Multivariable methods were not used for case-control studies until the late 1950s (Mantel and Haenszel, 1959). The first systematic treatment of the fourfold table and its inferential aspects in epidemiology was by Fleiss (1973). For example, consider the following hypothetical fourfold table:

	Characteristic Y		
Characteristic X	Present	Absent	Total
Present	A	B	A + B
Absent	C	D	C + C
Total	A + C	B + D	N = A + B + C + D

Inferences regarding the various parameters (cells) of this table depend on the method of sampling. If the table were produced by cross-sectional sampling (e.g., N attendees at a dinner are classified by sex and whether illness resulted), the methods for calculating estimates and significance levels would differ from those used if the sample design were purposive; that is, selection of a predetermined number of people who have characteristic X and for whom characteristic X is absent (see Chapter 2).

Developments and Controversies in Causality

Early observations on *causality* were made by the Romans in the first century B.C. regarding the relationship between swamps and disease (e.g., malaria) and the association of disease with occupation (e.g., protective mouthwear for flute players) (Rosen, 1958). Much of the later literature concerning causation was published in Europe in response to the plague epidemic (i.e., Black Death) in the mid-1300s (Rosen, 1958). At that time, the understanding of causality assumed that diseases were caused by an imbalance among the four humors: phlegm, blood, yellow bile, and black bile. Beyond this, the next enumeration of criteria for establishing causality has been attributed to Koch (Pinner and Pinner, 1932), who established the germ theory of disease by isolating and culturing the tuberculosis bacilli and producing the disease by subsequent inoculation into animals. These postulates involve establishing the strength of an association, a dose-response effect, the lack of temporal ambiguity, consistency of findings, biological plausibility of the hypothesis, coherence of the evidence, and specificity of the association (Hill, 1971).

   Correlations and other measures of association (e.g., risk estimates) are statistical estimates that can be used to establish only one of the criteria for causation (strength of association); it is a dangerous mistake to assume that correlation and causation are identical. An early discussion of the pitfalls of using correlations to infer causation is found in Yule's 1895 paper on poverty. One hundred years later, the term "lurking variable" was introduced as a precursor to confounding (Stigler, 1986). The term "confounding," coined by Sartwell (1981), refers to a characteristic associated (correlated) with both the risk factor of interest and the outcome, and proved especially useful in studying diseases with a long latent interval between exposure and onset (Susser, 1985) as well as newly identified infectious diseases (e.g., legionnaires disease [Fraser et al., 1977] and toxic shock syndrome [Langmuir, 1982]).

Criteria for evidence of causation (rather than correlation) in situations where ethical or logistic problems preclude experimentation were published by Hill (1965) and augmented in a quality-of-evidence scale by Donham and Thorn (1994). More recent work indicates that randomization as a means of validating causality has been oversold when used to evaluate social intervention programs. Several factors make causation difficult to assess. First, distinguishing correlation from causation is problematic (Petitti 1991; Goodman, 1994). Second, it is difficult to determine what constitutes a disease, rather than a marker for a disease (Medical Research Council Working Party, 1992). Third, it is difficult to decide on the appropriate disease model. For example, the intervention for a condition determined by a stochastic or random process is different from that for a disease caused by invasion of a microorganism or exposure to an environmental agent with a deterministic mechanism. Fourth, purely observational studies cannot prove or disprove causality. Koch's final argument to prove that the *Myco-bacterium tuberculosis* organism was causative of tuberculosis was to inject the bacillus into animals; germs should not be injected into humans. According to philosopher Karl Popper, a hypothesis cannot be proved but only disproved by solely observational studies (Sutter, 1996). Sutter would advocate using simultaneous equations methods such as path analysis (Goldberger and Duncan, 1973) or Rubin's causal model (Rubin, 1974).

Despite this controversy, the use of statistics in public health has yielded visible results (Gail, 1996), such as the causal link between smoking and lung cancer (Brownlee, 1965; Stolley, 1991). In 1964, the U.S. Surgeon General's Report (Centers for Disease Control, 1964) summarized 15 years of data concerning the prevalence of smoking and its effects in this country. The collection, analysis, and interpretation of these data formed the basis for policy decisions regulating the use of tobacco in the United States (Kessler, 1996). Decision makers used evidence of nicotine's effect on the brain and the central nervous system as well as surveillance data concerning the relationship between variations in nicotine content and those in adolescent smoking habits to argue that nicotine is in fact a drug intended to affect the structure or function of the body. The recent policy ruling of the Food and Drug Administration (FDA) contains strong measures to limit adolescents' access to tobacco products.

Methods from Other Sciences and Technology

Analytic methods from other areas of science will continue to provide new tools for public health researchers and practitioners. For example, the forecasting and modeling methods presented in this chapter would not have been so widely used in public health had it not been for the rapid development and implementation of microcomputers and associated software. The term *public health informatics* encompasses the application of information science, engineering, and technology to public health (Kilbourne, 1992). The purpose of this application is to facilitate effective and efficient collection of data that can be used in the rapid assessment of community health, the early identification of outbreaks, and the provision of timely guidelines for public health practice (Thacker and Stroup, 1997). In addition, *geographic information systems* will permit unprecedented surveillance of the environment and greater understanding of known and suspected associations between environmental conditions and human or animal health (Croner et al., 1996).

Economic methods have been used to assist public policy decision making since 1844 (Clemmer and Haddix, 1996). These methods have been incorporated into *prevention effectiveness* studies (Haddix et al., 1996) and are now used in public health to choose among competing interventions (Miller et al., 1996) or to set priorities in institutions with resource constraints (Mansergh et al., 1996). Finally, methods from molecular epidemiology and genetics are increasingly important to public health (Ou et al., 1992). For example, molecular biological methods can be used to demonstrate the relatedness of viruses, lead to early diagnosis (e.g., human immunodeficiency virus [HIV] infected infants), and can suggest the risk of new modes of transmission (e.g., HIV and maternal breastfeeding). Genetic screening can be used to determine predisposition to autoimmunity with important implications for vaccination programs.

Conclusion

Statistics and other quantitative methods provide the basis of quantification in public health.

> Most people are not natural-born statisticians. Left to our own devices, we are not very good at picking out patterns from a sea of noisy data. To put it another way, we are all too good at picking out nonexistent patterns that happen to suit our purposes. Statistical theory attacks both problems: it provides optimal methods for finding a real signal in a noisy background, and also provides strict checks against the overinterpretation of random patterns. (Efron and Tibshirani, 1993)

The application of these quantitative methods in public health has led to our ability to project the burden of AIDS (Brookmeyer, 1996), argue effectively to remove lead from gasoline in the United States (Annest et al., 1983), take advantage of varicella vaccine for our children (Lieu et al., 1994), and determine when to administer Bacille Calmette-Guérin (BCG) vaccine to protect against tuberculosis (Frost, 1933) (see Chapter 9).

Statistical methods are central to advances in clinical medicine and those that extend to a community of people (Matthews, 1995). The challenge to readers of this book is to recognize the importance of measurement in public health and to understand its meaning. Quantitative descriptions of populations, quantification of risks, measurement of uncertainty, and comparison of population groups are fundamental statistical techniques. This book will present these techniques in the context of the public health approach: defining the problem, identifying risk factors, developing and testing prevention strategies, and implementing prevention programs.

References

Annest J. L., J. L. Pirkle, D. Makuc, J. W. Neese, D. D. Bayse, M. G. Kovar. Chronological trend in blood lead levels between 1976 and 1980. *N. Engl. J. Med.* 308: 1373–1377, 1983.

Artzrouni, M. AIDS projections: how Farr out? [Letter]. *JAMA* 263:1522–1525, 1990.

Bregman, D. J., and A. D. Langmuir. Farr's law applied to AIDS projections. *JAMA* 263:1538–1539, 1990.

Breslow, N. E. Statistics in epidemiology: the case-control study. *J. Am. Stat. Assoc.* 91:14–28, 1996.

Broders, A. C. Squamous-cell epithelioma of the lip. A study of five hundered and thirty-seven cases. *JAMA* 74:656–664, 1920.

Brookmeyer, R. AIDS, epidemics, and statistics. *Biometrics* 52:781–796, 1996.

Brookmeyer, R., and M. H. Gail. Minimum size of the acquired immunodeficiency syndrome (AIDS) epidemic in the United States. *Lancet* 2:1320–1322, 1986.

Brookmeyer, R., and C. Quinn. Estimation of current HIV incidence rates from a cross-sectional survey using early diagnostic tests. *Am. J. Epidemiol.* 141:166–172, 1995.

Brownlee, K. A. A review of "smoking and health." *J. Amer. Stat. Assoc.* 60:722–739, 1965.

Budd, W. *Typhoid Fever: Its Nature, Mode of Spreading and Prevention.* New York: American Public Health Assocation, 1931.

Buehler, J. W., K. M. DeCock, and J. B. Brunet. Surveillance definitions for AIDS. *AIDS* 7(Suppl.):S73–S81, 1993.

Burchfield, R. W., (ed.). *A Supplement to the Oxford English Dictionary, A–G.* Oxford: Clarendon, 1972.

Canadian Task Force on the Periodic Health Examination. *The Canadian Guide to Clinical Preventive Health Care.* Ottawa: Canada Communication Group, 1994.

Centers for Disease Control. *Smoking and Health: Report of the Advisory Committee to the Surgeon General of the Public Health Service.* Atlanta, 1964.

Centers for Disease Control and Prevention. Rapid health needs assessment following Hurricane Andrew—Florida and Louisiana, 1992. *MMWR Morb. Mortal. Wkly. Rep.* 41:685–688, 1992.

Charlton, B.G. Should epidemiologists be pragmatists, biostatisticians, or clinical scientists? *Epidemiology* 7(5):552–554, 1996.

Clemmer, B., and A. Haddix. Cost-benefit analysis. In: *Prevention Effectiveness: A Guide to Decision Analysis and Economic Evaluation,* edited by A. C. Haddix, S. M. Teutsch, P. A. Shaffer, and D. O. Duñet. New York: Oxford University Press, 1996.

Cole, P. The evolving case-control study. *J. Chronic Dis.* 32:15–27, 1979.

Cornfield, J. A method of estimating comparative rates from clinical data. Applications to cancer of the lung, breast, and cervix. *J. Natl. Cancer Inst.* 11:1269–1275, 1951.

The Commission on Chronic Illness. *I. Prevention of Chronic Illness. 1956; II. Chronic Illness in the United States; Care of the Long-Term Patient. 1957; III. Chronic Illness in a Rural Area: The Hunterdon Study; 1958; IV. Chronic Illness in a Large City; 1959.* Cambridge, MA: Harvard University Press.

Croner, C. M, J. Sperling, and F. R. Broome. Geographic information systems (GIS): new perspectives in understanding human health and environmental relationships. *Stat. Med.* 15:1961–1977, 1996.

Davidson, R. A. Does it work or not? Clinical vs statistical significance. *Chest* 106:932–934, 1994.

Davies, N. *Europe: A History.* New York: Oxford University Press, 1996.

Dawber, T. R. *The Framingham Study: The Epidemiology of Coronary Heart Disease.* Cambridge, MA: Harvard University Press, 1980.

Deming, W. E., and A. Stuart. Sample surveys. In: *International Encyclopedia of Statistics.* London: Collier Macmillan, 1968.

Donham, K. F., and P. S. Thorne. Agents in organic dust: criteria for a causal relationship. *Am. J. Ind. Med.* 25:33–39, 1994.

Dwyer, J. H., and M. Feinleib. Report of a workshop on statistical issues in longitudinal studies of health. *Stat. Med.* 7:177–183, 1988.

Efron, B., and R. Tibshirani. *An Introduction to the Bootstrap.* New York: Chapman & Hall, 1993.

Ethridge, E. *Sentinel for Health.* Berkeley, CA: University of California Press, 1992.

Farley, D. O., T. Richards, R. M. Bell, and the Physician Payment Review Commission. Effects of reporting methods on infant mortality rate estimates for racial and ethnic subgroups. *Health Care Poor Underserved* 6:60–75, 1995.

Farr, W. The provincial medical and surgical association. *Br. Ann. Med.* 1:692–695, 1837.

Fechner, G. T. *Elemente der Psychophysik,* 2 Vols. Vol. 1, edited by D. H. Howes and E. G. Boring [German]. New York: Holt, Rinehart & Winston, 1860.

Fee, E. *Disease and Discovery: History of the Johns Hopkins School of Hygiene and Public Health, 1916–1939.* Baltimore, MD: The Johns Hopkins University Press, 1987.

Feinleib, M. Counting isn't easy. [Editorial]. *Epidemiology* 6:343–345, 1995.

Fisher, R. A. *Statistical Methods for Research Workers.* Edinburgh: Oliver & Boyd, 1925.

Fisher, R. A. The arrangement of field experiments. *J. Ministry Agriculture Great Britain* 33:503–513, 1926.

Fleiss, J. *Statistical Methods for Rates and Proportions.* New York: John Wiley & Sons, 1973.

Foege, W. H., R. C. Hogan, and L. H. Newton. Surveillance projects for selected diseases. *Int. J. Epidemiol.* 5:29–37, 1976.

Fraser, D. W., T. R.Tsai, W.Orenstein, et al. Legionnaires' disease: description of an epidemic of pneumonia. *N. Engl. J. Med.* 297:1189–1197, 1977.

Frost, W. H. Risk of persons in familial contact with pulmonary tuberculosis. *Am. J. Public Health* 23:426–432, 1933. In: *Papers of Wade Hampton Frost,* edited be K. F. Maxcy. New York: The Commonwealth Fund, 1941.

Gail, M. H. Statistics in action. *J. Amer. Stat. Assoc.* 91:1–13, 1996.

Gail, M. H., and R. Brookmeyer. Projecting the incidence of AIDS. *JAMA* 263:1538–1539, 1990.

Goldberger, A. S., and O. D. Duncan (Eds.). *Structural Equation Models in the Social Sciences.* New York: Academic Press, 1973.

Goldberger, J., G. A. Wheeler, and E. Sydenstricker. A study of the diet of non-pellagrous and pellagrous households in textile mill communities in South Carolina in 1916. *JAMA* 71:944–949, 1918.

Goodman, S. N. P values, hypothesis tests, and likelihood: implications for epidemiology of a neglected historical debate. *Am. J. Epidemiol.* 139:116–118, 1994.

Graunt, J. *Natural and Political Observations Mentioned in a Following Index, and Made upon the Bills of Mortality,* 3rd ed. London: John Martyn and James Allestry, 1665.

Greenberg, R. S., and D. G. Kleinbaum. Mathematical modeling strategies for the analysis of epidemiologic research. Ann. Rev. Public Health 6:223–245, 1985.

Greenwood, M. *Some British Pioneers of Social Medicine.* London: Oxford University Press, 1948.

Gross, M. Oswego County revisited. *Public Health Rep.* 91:168–169, 1976.

Haddix, A. C., S. M. Teutsch, P. A. Shaffer, and D. O. Dunet. *Prevention Effectiveness: A Guide to Decision Analysis and Economic Evaluation.* New York: Oxford University Press, 1996.

Haggett, P., A. D. Cliff, and A. Frey. *Locational Analysis in Human Geography,* 2nd edition. London: Edward Arnold Press, 1977.

Hahn, R. A., and S. Eberhardt. Life expectancy in four U. S. racial/ethnic populations. *Epidemiology* 6:350–355, 1990.

Hanzlick, R. Survey of medical examiner office computerization. From the National Association of Medical Examiners (N.A.M.E.). *Am. J. Forensic Med. Pathol.* 15:110–117, 1994.

Hill, A. B. The environment and disease: association or causation? *Proc. R. Soc. Med.* 58:295–300, 1965.

Hill, A. B. *Principles of Medical Statistics,* 9th ed. New York: Oxford University Press, 1971.

Houweling, H., and R. A. Coutinho. Acquired immunodeficiency syndrome. In *Oxford Textbook of Public Health,* 3rd ed. edited by R. Detels, W. W. Holland, J. McEwen, and G. S. Omenn. New York: Oxford University Press, 1997.

Irvine, P. W., N. Van Buren, and K. Crossley. Causes for hospitalization of nursing home residents: the role of infection. *J. Am. Geriatr. Soc.* 32:103–107, 1984.

Israel, R. A. Automation of mortality data coding and processing in the United States of America. *World Health Stat. Q.* 43:259–262, 1990.

Kahn, H. A., and C. T. Sempos. *Statistical Methods in Epidemiology.* New York: Oxford University Press, 1989.

Kendall, M. G., and A. Stuart. *The Advanced Theory of Statistics,* Vol. I. New York: Harner Publishing Company, 1969.

Kessler, D. A. *FDA's Regulation of Tobacco.* Presented at Centers for Disease Control and Prevention, Atlanta, Ga., November 6, 1996.

Kilbourne, E. M. Informatics in public health surveillance: current issues and future perspectives. In: *Proceedings of the 1992 International Symposium on Public Health Surveillance,* edited by S. F. Wetterhall. *MMWR Morbid. Mortal. Wkly. Rep.* 41(Suppl): S91–S99, 1992.

Lambert, R. *Sir John Simon (1816–1904) and English Social Administration.* London: MacGibbon and Kee, 1963.

Lancaster, H. O. *Expectations of Life: A Study in the Demography, Statistics, and History of World Mortality.* New York: Springer-Verlag, 1990.

Lane-Claypon, J. E. A further report on cancer of the breast. *Reports on Public Health and Medical Subjects, Ministry of Health.* London: Her Majesty's Stationery Office, 1926.

Langmuir, A. D. The surveillance of communicable diseases of national importance. *N. Engl. J. Med.* 288:182–192, 1963.

Langmuir, A. D. William Farr: founder of modern concepts of surveillance. *Int. J. Epidemiol.* 5:13–18, 1976.

Langmuir, A. D. Toxic shock syndrome: an epidemiologist's viewpoint. *J. Infect. Dis.* 145:588–591, 1982.

Langmuir, A. D. The territory of epidemiology: pentimento. *J. Infect. Dis.* 155:349–358, 1987.

Laplace, P. S. 1786. Sur les naissances, les mariages et les morts, à Paris, depuis 1771 jusqui'en 1784, et dans toute l'étendue de la France, pendant les années 1781 and 1782. *Mémoires de l'Académie Royale des Sciences de Paris,* 1783.

Legendre, A. M. *Nouvelles méthodes pour la détermination des orbites des comètes* [French] . Paris: Courcier, 1805.

Levin, M. L., H. Goldstein, and P. R. Gerhardt. Cancer and tobacco smoking: a preliminary report. *JAMA* 143:336–338, 1950.

Lexis, W. *Zur Theorie der Massenerscheinungen in der Menschlichen Gesellschaft.* [German]. Freiburg: Wagner, 1877.

Lieu, T. A., S. B. Black, N. Rieser, P. Ray, E. M. Lewis, and H. R. Shinefield. The cost of childhood chickenpox: parents' perspective. *Pediatr. Infect. Dis. J.* 13:173–177, 1994.

Lilienfeld, A. M., and D. E. Lilienfeld. A century of case-control studies: progress? *J. Chronic. Dis.* 32:5–13, 1979.

Lind, J. A treatise of the scurvy in three parts: containing an inquiry into the nature, causes, and cure of that disease together with a critical and chronological view of what has been published on the subject. In: *Lind's Treatise on Scurvy,* edited by C. P. Stewart and D. Guthrie. Edinburgh: Churchill, 1953.

Lombard, H. L., and C. R. Doering. Cancer studies in Massachusetts. 2. Habits, characteristics and environment of individuals with and without cancer. *N. Engl. J. Med.* 198:481–487, 1928.

Louis, P. C. A. *Researches on the Effects of Bloodletting in Some Inflammatory Diseases, and on the Influence of Tartarized Antimony and Vesication in Pneumonitis.* Boston: Milliard, Gray and Co., 1836.

Lui, K. J., D. N. Lawrence, W. M. Morgan, et al. A model based approach for estimating the mean incubation period of transfusion-associated acquired immunodeficiency syndrome. *Proc. Nat. Acad. Sci. U.S.A.* 83:3051–3055, 1986.

MacMahon, B., T. F. Pugh, and J. Ipsen. *Epidemiological Methods.* Boston: Little, Brown & Co., 1960.

Mansergh, G., A. Haddix, R. Steketee, et al. Cost-effectiveness of short-course zidovudine to present perinatal HIV in developing country settings. *JAMA* 276:139–145, 1996.

Mantel, N., and W. Haenszel. Statistical aspects of data from retrospective studies of disease. *J. Natl. Cancer. Inst.* 22:719–748, 1959.

Matthews, J. R. *Quantification and the Quest for Medical Certainty.* Princeton, NJ: Princeton University Press, 1995.

Medical Research Council Working Party. Medical Research Council trial of treatment of hypertension in older adults: principal results. *Br. Med. J.* 304:405–412, 1992.

Miller, M. A., R. W. Sutter, P. M. Strebel, and S. C. Hadler. Cost-effectiveness of incorporating inactivated poliovirus vaccine into the routine childhood immunization schedule. *JAMA* 276:967–971, 1996.

Mundlak, Y. Cross-section analysis. In: *International Encyclopedia of Statistics,* edited by J. Tanur, and W. Kruskal. New York: Macmillan, 1978; pp. 90–95.

Murray, J. D. *Mathematical Biology,* 2nd ed. New York: Springer, 1993.

Ohadike, D. C. Diffusion and physiological responses to the influenza pandemic of 1918–19 in Nigeria. *Soc. Sci. Med.* 32:1393–1399, 1991.

Ou, C. Y., C. A. Ciesielski, G. Myers, et al. Molecular epidemiology of HIV transmission in a dental practice. *Science* 256:1165–1171, 1992.

Petitti, D. B. Associations are not effects. *Am. J. Epidemiol.* 133:101–102, 1991.

Pierce, C. S., and J. Jastrow. On small differences of sensation. *Mem. Nat. Acad. Sci.* 3:75–83, 1885.

Pinner, B., and M. Pinner. The aetiology of tuberculosis. *Am. Rev. Tuberculosis* 25:285–323, 1932.

Quetelet, L. A. J. Recherches sur la population, les naissances, les décès, les prisons, les dépôs, de mendicité, etc., dan le royaume des Pays-Bas [French]. *Nouveaux mémoires de l'Académie Royale des Sciences et Belles-lettres de Bruxelles* 4:117–192, 1827.

Quetelet, L. A. J. *Instructions populaires sur le calcul des probabilités* [French]. Brussels: Tarlier et Hayez, 1828.

Quetelet, L. A. J. *Sur l'homme et le développement de ses facultés, ou Essai de physique sociale* [French]. Paris: Bachelier, 1835.

Rice, D. P. Health statistics: past and present. [Editorial]. *N. Engl. J. Med.* 305:219–220, 1981.

Robins, J. M., and S. Greenland. The role of model selection in causal inference from non-experimental data. *Am. J. Epidemiol.* 123:392–402, 1986.

Rose, G. Sick individuals and sick populations. *Int. J. Epidemiol.* 14:32–38, 1985.

Rosen, G. *A History of Public Health.* New York: MD Publications, Inc., 1958.

Rubin, D. B. Estimating causal effects of treatment in randomized and nonrandomized studies. *J. Educ. Psychol.* 66:688–701, 1974.

Rvachev, L. A., and I. M. Longini. A mathematical model for the global spread of influenza. *Math. Biosci.* 75:3–22, 1985.

Sartwell, P. E. Infectious hepatitis in relation to blood tranfusion. *Bull. U. S. Army Med. Dep.* 7:90–100, 1947.

Sartwell, P. E. The distribution of incubation periods of infectious diseases. *Am. J. Hygiene* 51:310–318, 1950.

Sartwell, P. E. Retrospective studies: a view for the clinician. *Ann. Intern. Med.* 94:381–386, 1981.

Schnell, D., A. Zaidi, and G. Reynolds. A time series analysis of gonorrhea surveillance data. *Stat. Med.* 8:343–352, 1989.

Schreck, R., L. A. Baker, G. P. Ballard, and S. Dolgoff. Tobacco smoking as an etiologic factor in disease: I. Cancer. Cancer Res. 10:49–58, 1950.

Schreck, R., and H. Lenowitz. Etiologic factors in carcinoma of the penis. *Cancer Res.* 7:180–187, 1947.

Serfling, R. E., and I. L. Sherman. *Attribute Sampling Methods for Local Health Departments with Special Reference to Immunization Surveys.* Washington, DC: United States Government Printing Office, Publication No. 1230, 1965.

Shakespeare, E. O. *Report on Cholera in Europe and India.* Washington, DC: Government Printing Office, 1890.

Shattuck, L. *Report of a General Plan for the Promotion of Public and Personal Health Devised, Prepared and Recommended by the Commissioners Appointed under a Resolve of the Legislature of Massachusetts Relating to a Sanitary Survey of the State.* Boston, MA: Dutton and Wentworth. Cambridge, MA: Harvard University Press, 1848.

Shy, C. M. The failure of academic epidemiology: witness for the prosecution. *Am. J. Epidemiol.* 145:479–487, 1997.

Simon, J. *English Sanitary Institutions.* London: Cassell, 1890.

Sladen, B. K., and F. B. Bang (Eds). *Biology of Populations: The Biological Basis of Public Health.* New York: American Elsevier, 1969.

Snow, J. On the mode of communication of cholera. In: *Snow on Cholera.* New York: The Commonwealth Fund, 1936, pp. 1–175.

Stigler, S. M. *The History of Statistics: The Measurement of Uncertainty Before 1900.* Cambridge: Harvard University Press, 1986.

Stolley, P. D. When genius errs: R. A. Fisher and the lung cancer controversy. *Am. J. Epidemiol.* 133:416–428, 1991.

Stroup, D. F., S. B. Thacker, and J. L. Herndon. Application of multiple time series analysis to the estimation of pneumonia and influenza mortality by age: 1962–1983. *Stat. Med.* 7:1045–1059, 1988.

Stroup, D. F., G. D. Williamson, J. L. Herndon, and J. M. Karon. Detection of aberrations in the occurrence of notifiable diseases surveillance data. *Stat. Med.* 8:323–329, 1989.

Suits, D. B. Use of dummy variables in regression equations. *J. Am. Stat. Assoc.* 52:548–551, 1957.

Susser, M. Epidemiology in the United States after World War II: the evolution of technique. *Epidemiol. Rev.* 7:147–177, 1985.

Sutter, M. C. Assigning causation in disease: beyond Koch's postulates. *Perspect. Biol. Med.* 39:581–592, 1996.

Taubes, G. Epidemiology faces its limits. *Science* 269:164–169, 1995.

Thacker, S. B. The principles and practice of public health surveillance: use of data in public health practice. *Sante Publique* 4:43–49, 1992.

Thacker, S. B., and M. B. Gregg. Implementing the concepts of William Farr: the contributions of Alexander D. Langmuir to public health surveillance and communications. *Am. J. Epidemiol.* 144:S23–S28, 1996.

Thacker, S. B., and J. D. Millar. Mathematical modeling and attempts to eliminate measles: a tribute to the late Professor George Macdonald. *Am. J. Epidemiol.* 133:517–525, 1991.

Thacker, S.B., and D. F. Stroup. Persistence of influenza A by continuous close-contact transmission: the effect of non-random mixing. *Int. J. Epidemiol.* 10:1078–1082, 1990.

Thacker, S. B., and D. F. Stroup. Future directions of comprehensive public health surveillance and health information systems in the United States. *Am. J. Epidemiol.* 140:383–397, 1994.

Thacker, S. B., and D. F. Stroup. Public health surveillance. In: *Applied Epidemiology,* edited by R. C. Brownson, and D. P. Petitti. New York: Oxford University Press, 1997.

Thompson, W. D. Effect modification and the limits of biological inference from epidemiologic data. *J. Clin. Epidemiol.* 44:221–232, 1991.

Velleman, P. F., and D. C. Hoaglin. *Applications, Basics, and Computing of Exploratory Data Analysis.* Boston: Duxbury Press, 1981.

Winslow, C. A., W. G. Smillie, J. A. Doull, and J. E. Gordon. *The History of American Epidemiology.* St. Louis: The CV Mosby Company, 1952.

Wright, S. The application of path analysis to etiology. In: *Genetic Epidemiology,* edited by N. E. Morton, and C. S. Chung. New York: Academic Press, 1978.

Wynder, E. L., and E. A. Graham. Tobacco smoking as a possible etiologic factor in bronchiogenic carcinoma. *JAMA* 143:329–338, 1950.

Yule, G. U. On the correlation of total pauperism with proportion of out-relief, I: all ages. *Econ. J.* 5:603–611, 1885.

Zaidi, A., D. Schnell, and G. Reynolds. A time series analysis of syphilis surveillance data. *Stat. Med.* 8:251–400, 1989.

2

Basic Concepts of Statistics

NANCY D. BARKER

> The theory of probabilities is at bottom nothing but common sense reduced to calculus.
> —Pierre Simon de Laplace 1749–1827

A genuine understanding of basic statistical concepts is critical for applying appropriate quantitative methods to public health practice. From the epidemiologist trying to determine the source of illness in an outbreak investigation to the physician interpreting the results from a statistical analysis in a medical journal, this core knowledge is imperative. Basic understanding of statistical concepts is becoming more essential with increasing technology and software development. Although a novice can perform the most sophisticated statistical techniques with a simple keystroke, quantitative methods may be inappropriately used by those who are not familiar with important details of the statistical techniques and nuances of any software used (e.g., neglecting to account for the survey design in the analysis of data from complex sample surveys).

Persons who analyze, interpret, and use quantitative information must understand key concepts of statistics. This chapter provides the reader with a description of the fundamental concepts of statistics that are important for solving practical public health problems.

Role of Randomness

Quantitative methods used in the analysis of public health data are founded on *probability theory*. Probability has long been associated with games of chance. In the late 1800s, scientific researchers began to consider that the same theory involving uncertainty in games of chance was related to the uncertainty in the outcomes in their own fields of study (Giri, 1993). Originally, disease processes were considered to be *deterministic* (i.e., scientists believed that if all the variables related to the disease could be controlled or were known, then the outcome could be predicted with certainty). The deliberation that disease outcomes follow a *stochastic* or random pattern rather than a deterministic one opened up a new field to the scientific community and contributed to the role of probability as being indispensable in the field of epidemiology and public health (see Chapter 1).

Probability also provides the foundation for *statistical inference,* or drawing conclusions about an entire *population* from information obtained about a *sample* from that population (see the section Significance Testing and Confidence Interval Estimation, later in this chapter). Probability is indispensable in the field of statistics. Entire books have been written to describe its theory and applications (Giri, 1993; Daniel, 1995; Williams, 1993).

Characteristics of a Frequency Distribution

Public health officials are provided with large amounts of information daily. This information must be summarized to help direct public health action and policy. The following example illustrates the use of a histogram for summarizing the incubation time periods for 43 cases of hepatitis A (Fig. 2.1). A *histogram* is a graph of a frequency distribution. Data should be examined graphically before trying to summarize them with a single summary measure (e.g., a mean). This visual presentation facilitates identification of outliers and examination of the shape of the distribution.

Two important properties of a frequency distribution are *central tendency* and

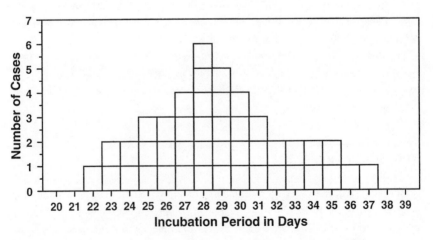

Figure 2.1. Hepatitis A cases by incubation period in days, sample city, 1992.

variation, or *dispersion.* The shape (symmetrical or skewed) of the distribution helps to determine the most appropriate measure of central tendency and dispersion.

A measure of central tendency is a single summary measure used to characterize the data. The most common measure of central tendency is the *arithmetic mean.* The Greek letter mu (μ) represents the mean of a population. A summary measure of a population is called a parameter. The formula for the population mean is:

$$\mu = \frac{\sum x_i}{N}$$

where x_i are the observations from the whole population. The symbol $\bar{x}$ denotes the mean of a sample from a population. Summary values of a sample are called statistics. The formula for the sample mean is:

$$\bar{x} = \frac{\sum x_i}{n}$$

where x_i are the observations from the sample. The mean is extremely sensitive to outliers and therefore may be most useful for data sets that are approximately symmetrical. The mean incubation time period for the 43 cases of hepatitis A described above is 1244/43 or 28.9 days.

The *median* is another common measure of central tendency that is useful in public health. The median is the middle value of the distribution. The median position is calculated, and that value is used to determine the median of the distribution.

$$\text{Median position} = \frac{n+1}{2}$$

The median is less affected by extreme or outlying values than is the mean, and, therefore, is often the preferred measure of central tendency for skewed distributions. The median position for the hepatitis A data is 22; therefore, the median incubation time period is 29 days.

The third and least common measure of central tendency is the *mode.* It is the value that occurs most often in the distribution, or that value with the highest frequency. The mode of the hepatitis A data is 28 days.

In this example, the three measures of central tendency yield similar results. This is characteristic of symmetrical distributions. Due to the mathematical properties that the mean possesses, the mean is the preferred measure for symmetrical distributions.

A single summary measure (e.g., a measure of central tendency) usually is not sufficient for characterizing a distribution, because it does not reflect the second important characteristic of a frequency distribution—its variation or dispersion. The *range* is the simplest measure of dispersion to compute. However, because it is extremely sensitive to outliers, it is the least useful. The range is equal to the largest value minus the smallest value. In the previously illustrated hepatitis A example, the range is $37 - 22$, or 15 days.

A second measure of dispersion is the *variance*. The variance is an average of the squared deviations from the mean. The square of the Greek letter sigma (σ^2) represents the population variance. The sample variance is represented by s^2. The following formulas define the population and the sample variances:

$$\text{Population:} \quad \sigma^2 = \frac{\Sigma (x_i - \mu)^2}{N}$$

$$\text{Sample:} \quad s^2 = \frac{\Sigma (x_i - \bar{x})^2}{n - 1}$$

where N is the total number in the population, and n is the total number in the sample. The variance of the sample of 43 incubation time periods in the above example is 13.5. The *standard deviation* (s), which is the square root of the variance, is 3.7.

The relationship between the mean and the standard deviation is important. The empirical rule states that given a set of n measurements that are approximately normally distributed, then, on average, the interval $\bar{x} \pm s$ contains 68.3% of the measurements, the interval $\bar{x} \pm 2s$ contains 95.5% of the measurements, and the interval $\bar{x} \pm 3s$ contains 99.7% of the measurements (Fig. 2.2).

Note that the interval $\bar{x} \pm 1.96s$ contains 95% of the measurements (see section Significance Testing and Confidence Interval Estimation, later in this chapter). Moore and McCabe (1989) provide a complete discussion of properties of frequency distributions.

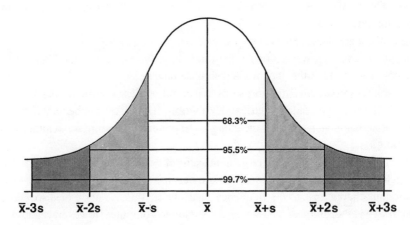

Figure 2.2. Bell curve demonstrating the relationship between the mean and the standard deviation.

Measurement of Risk

The three most common measures of disease frequency are ratios, proportions, and rates. A *ratio* is an expression of the relationship of any two quantities. Although the two quantities need not be related, they commonly are (e.g., the number of infant deaths in a particular year to the number of live births in the same year). A proportion is a ratio in which the numerator is included in the denominator, such as the number of women living in the United States who develop breast cancer in a particular year over the total number of women in the United States. A *rate* is the most common measure of disease frequency used in epidemiology. A true rate is a change per unit time. Some of the rates used in epidemiology are not true rates, but rather proportions. These terms are often misused in epidemiology (Elandt-Johnson, 1975).

The frequency measures described in this section can be categorized into two groups: prevalence and incidence. *Prevalence* measures the number of existing cases of disease, whereas incidence measures only the number of new cases of disease over a specified time interval. *Incidence* is typically used for presenting infectious diseases or those with short duration. Prevalence estimates the burden of a disease on a population and is most often used for chronic diseases or those infectious diseases with long durations. There are two important types of incidence. The first is *cumulative incidence,* which is actually a proportion (although commonly referred to as a rate) that describes the risk of illness for persons in a population. Cumulative incidence is the number of new cases in a defined population over a specified period of time divided by the population at risk during the same time period. For example, in the church supper outbreak in Oswego, NY (Gross, 1976), 46 of the 75 guests interviewed developed a gastrointestinal illness. The cumulative incidence is 46/75, or 61%. The cumulative incidence for such a short defined period is an *attack rate*. The cumulative incidence is a measure of risk for members in a population. Those attending the picnic had a 61% chance of becoming ill.

The second measure of incidence is actually a true rate called the *incidence density rate.* This rate is the number of new cases in a defined population over a specified period of time divided by the total amount of time each person was followed or observed totaled for all persons in the population of interest. For example, in a classic study by Doll and Hill (1964a,b), the incidence density rate for lung cancer mortality among smokers was 133 lung cancer–related deaths of 102,600 person-years at risk, or 1.30 cases per 1000 person-years. Unlike the cumulative incidence, the incidence density does not indicate the risk for an individual in a population; it represents the rate at which new cases are occurring. The incidence density utilizes more specific information regarding the members of a population because it uses the amount of time each subject was observed. This is particularly useful in follow-up studies where many persons are lost to follow-up and some are followed longer than others. The denominators of both of these measures of incidence need to be considered carefully. Only those who are at risk for the disease should be included in the calculation.

Period prevalence is also a proportion (commonly referred to as a rate) and is defined as the number of existing cases of disease in a population over a specified time interval divided by the population at risk during the same time interval. Point prevalence is the same as the period prevalence for a specific point in time rather than a time interval.

Measures of association are useful for assessing whether a relationship exists between exposure to a particular risk factor and disease status. The appropriate measure of association depends on the study design employed. For cohort studies, the most commonly used measure of association is the *relative risk*. The relative risk (occasionally referred to as a *risk ratio*) is a ratio of the attack rates in the exposed and unexposed groups. A relative risk of 1 indicates that the rates are the same in the two groups. A relative risk of above 1 indicates that those exposed are more likely to become ill. A relative risk of below 1 indicates that those unexposed are more likely to become ill (i.e., a protective effect). For example, in the Oswego study previously described, the data regarding the exposure status for one exposure and corresponding outcome for the 75 interviewed guests can be summarized in the following 2 × 2 table.

	Ill	Well	Totals
Exposed	43	11	54
Not Exposed	3	18	21
Totals	46	29	75

The attack rate in the exposed group is 43/54, or 80%. The attack rate in the unexposed group is 3/21, or 14%. The relative risk for the exposed group versus the unexposed group is 80%/14%, or 5.7, which means that the risk for illness in the exposed group was 5.7 times the risk in the unexposed group. Statistical tests can be performed to determine if this observed association is significantly different than 1 (i.e., no effect) (Fleiss, 1982).

The *risk difference* is another measure of association used in cohort studies. The difference in the attack rates of the exposed and unexposed groups is calculated to determine if it is significantly different from zero (i.e., no effect).

The *rate ratio* is a third measure of association used in cohort studies. It is the ratio of two incidence density rates and is useful when the person-time information is available. The interpretation is similar to that for the relative risk.

Because disease rates typically are not available in case-control studies, the *odds ratio* is the commonly used measure of association. The odds ratio is the ratio of the odds of exposure among cases and controls. In the following table, the odds ratio is calculated by determining the odds of exposure among the cases (a/c) divided by the odds of exposure among controls (b/d).

	Case	Control
Exposed	a	b
Not Exposed	c	d

The common formula for calculating the odds ratio is ad/bc. If the disease is rare, then the odds ratio closely approximates the relative risk (Schlesselman, 1982). The interpretation of the odds ratio is similar to that of the relative risk (i.e., an odds ratio above 1 indicates that the relationship of the disease to exposure is unlikely to be due to chance).

Another important issue regarding rates is *rate adjustment.* When comparing rates of disease among two or more populations with different age distributions (e.g., Alaska and Florida), one population may have a higher rate than the other. This difference may not be indicative of increased risk, but indicative of a higher proportion of persons in an age group in one *population* that may be *related to* the frequency of the disease. In this situation, adjusting or standardizing the rates to remove the effect of age and make them comparable is sometimes useful.

Age standardization is a method that controls for age as a factor. The rate in the population of interest can be standardized several ways depending on what information is available. Fleiss (1981) describes direct and indirect methods for rate standardization. Direct standardization is preferred unless data needed for calculation are lacking or small numbers of events make rates unstable. Standardized rates have no meaning in isolation; they can only be used to compare with some other rate standardized in the same way.

Basic Concepts of Sampling

Surveys often are conducted to find the answer to a question of public health importance. Surveying everyone in a population of interest often is not practical or economically feasible; therefore, a *sample* is selected as representative of that population. The goal is to make inferences from the sample to the population; the population actually surveyed must closely match the population of interest. For example, in a survey of women's attitudes regarding day care, it would not be a good strategy to conduct door-to-door surveys during working hours—the accessible population (i.e., women with preschool children at home during working hours) would not represent the target population (i.e., all women with preschool children).

When designing surveys, the difference between probability and nonprobability samples should be understood. A *probability sample* is one in which each element in a population has a known and nonzero probability of being included in the sample (Kish, 1965). An example of a nonprobability sample is a *convenience sample* (e.g., sampling everyone in three counties to represent the entire state). The elements in the other counties have no probability of inclusion in the study. Sampling distribution theory is developed for analyzing data from probability samples. Statistical analysis accounts for sampling errors. However, nonsampling errors cannot be controlled with statistics, and the effect these errors have on the estimates cannot be determined.

Four types of probability samples are used most often in epidemiology. A *simple random sample* (SRS) is the easiest type of sample to understand. A sample of size *n* is randomly selected from a population of size *N*. Each sample of size *n* has the same probability *n/N* of inclusion. A SRS is appealing not only because it is easy to understand but because it is easy to analyze. Most standard statistical software packages are designed to analyze data from an SRS. An SRS often is not practical, however, because the required sampling frame frequently is large or disperse. Getting a list of all elements in the population may not even be possible. In addition, an SRS may not be economical in some cases because of geographic dispersion of the sample in large populations. However, an SRS often is used as one of several stages in the selection of a probability sample.

The SRS and the *systematic sample* are similarly designed. A systematic sample also requires a list of the population as the sampling frame; however, the random selection is done by obtaining a random start, then selecting every k^{th} element that is based on the desired sample size ($k = N/n$). The systematic sample is easier and faster to implement than the SRS. The systematic sample works well and can be analyzed as an SRS when the population list has no inherent order that could create bias.

A third important probability sample is the *stratified random sample*. A stratified sample survey is accomplished by dividing the population into appropriate nonoverlapping strata and selecting a probability sample within each stratum. This design is appropriate when (*1*) the elements tend to be similar within strata with respect to the outcome of interest and (*2*) the elements from different strata are very different from one another. For example, children in the same age groups (i.e., strata) tend to be similar with respect to vaccine status (i.e., outcome), and children in different age groups tend to differ from one another with respect to vaccine status. When the variation within groups is less than the variation among groups, the stratified design will yield smaller variances than will the SRS.

The fourth probability sample often used in public health worldwide is the *cluster sample*. Cluster sampling frequently is used in public health surveys when the travel and personnel costs associated with conducting surveys are determining factors. When using a cluster design, the population is divided into groups, or clusters, of elements (i.e., sampling units). A sample of clusters is selected from the population and either all or a sample of elements from the clusters is included in the study. Unlike stratified sampling, the maximum benefits of cluster sampling are achieved when the entire population is well mixed (either naturally or by the researcher) so that clusters are very different within but alike from cluster to cluster with respect to the outcome of interest. Unfortunately, this often does not occur in practice. For example, when selecting city blocks or villages as clusters, persons living in close proximity may be more alike with respect to attitude toward preventive care than those living in different clusters. In cluster sampling, this type of association may actually increase the variance. One advantage to cluster sampling is that once clusters are selected, only a list of all the elements from the selected clusters is needed, which can substantially reduce time and expense.

Multistage surveys incorporate several of these probability sample strategies together. For example, suppose a study is planned in which parents of school children are to be surveyed about their attitudes regarding handguns. One strategy for selecting this sample may be to first select school children and then to survey their parents. The population may be divided into rural and urban school districts (i.e., strata). Then schools may be randomly selected as clusters of children (i.e., primary sampling unit, or the first stage of random selection) from the rural and urban districts. Then, within each selected school, classrooms may be randomly selected, and each child in the selected classroom would be included in the study. This method of obtaining the sample is only one of many possible methods. It is important to consider the best way to allocate or distribute the sample (see Scheaffer et al., 1986). The probabilities of selection must be noted at every stage of the design, especially when unequal probabilities of selection are used (e.g., oversampling a particular subgroup to ensure adequate representation). *Weights* must be used when the probabilities of selection differ for the elements in the survey. A *sampling weight* is defined as the inverse of the probability of selection. The sum of the sample weights of the selected elements should equal the total population size (Cochran, 1977; Kish, 1965).

Survey design (including weights when required) must be taken into account when analyzing data from a complex sample survey. Researchers often conduct elaborate survey designs and then analyze the data as if they were from a simple random sample. Results obtained without taking design into account often differ from results obtained after accounting for the design—thus yielding potentially misleading results.

The *design effect* (DEFF) should be considered when contemplating complex sample surveys. The DEFF can be quantified as the variance from the design divided by the variance assuming an SRS and is a measure of the efficiency of the design. The DEFF answers the question, "What is lost (or gained) by conducting the survey using a particular design relative to an SRS?" If the DEFF is equal to 1, the variance incorporating the design and the variance assuming an SRS are the same; the results should be the same as results obtained assuming an SRS. If the

DEFF is above 1 (i.e., the variance accounting for the design is larger than that for an SRS), and the design is not accounted for in the analysis, the researcher may erroneously conclude that a significant effect exists, when in fact, it does not. This type of assumption constitutes a type I error (see section Significance Testing and Confidence Interval Estimation, later in this chapter). If the design effect is below 1 (i.e., the variance from the design is smaller than that for an SRS), researchers would be less likely to detect a significant effect, which constitutes a type II error.

The following example illustrates how one might obtain misleading results by not accounting for design. In a recent disaster survey that employed a two-stage cluster design (Centers for Disease Control and Prevention, 1993), the proportion of the population with a certain characteristic was estimated to be 66.8% (95% confidence interval = 55.7%, 78.0%). These estimates accounted for the two-stage cluster design employed. If the analysis had ignored the design and these data were treated as if from an SRS, the point estimate would have remained the same in this unweighted design (66.8%); however, the corresponding 95% confidence interval would have been inappropriately too narrow (61.2%, 72.5%). Based on the correct variance from the complex design, this interval corresponds to only a 67% confidence interval. Not accounting for the design in this analysis would provide results that are not only inappropriate, but misleading.

Lack of readily accessible, easy-to-use software has probably been the biggest reason for not accounting for the design of complex sample surveys. Standard software packages do not provide appropriate variances for such complex designs. Recently, however, several packages have addressed this problem. EPI-INFO provides a module called CSAMPLE designed to analyze such data (Dean et al., 1993). SUDAAN is a very powerful tool for analyzing such data and can perform statistical modeling (Shah et al., 1991).

Significance Testing and Confidence Interval Estimation

Typically in public health, a sample is obtained from a defined population that is described using summary measures (e.g., mean, median, mode, relative risk, and odds ratio). These measures are included in a branch of statistics called *descriptive statistics*. *Inferential statistics* is that branch of statistics that facilitates making generalizations to a population from information obtained in a sample from that population. This section on significance testing and confidence interval estimation provides the necessary background for making inference to populations from data obtained from a sample. The hepatitis A example described earlier illustrates the theory behind the test of significance and the estimation of a confidence interval for a mean.

When conducting significance testing, a null and alternative hypothesis must be determined. The *null hypothesis* (H_o) and *alternative hypothesis* (H_a) are set up to seek sufficient evidence that the null hypotheses is false and reject it in favor of the alternative. In the hepatitis A example given in a previous section (titled Characteristics of a Frequency Distribution), suppose that the average incubation time period in this hypothetical population is considered to be 27 days. The hypothesis that the incubation time period is not equal to 27 days can be tested using the sample of 43.

A *test of significance* can yield one of four results. The following table summarizes these events.

		Your Decision	
		Accept H_o	Reject H_o
	Accept H_o	√	Type I error (α)
Truth			
	Reject H_o	Type II error (β)	√ (Power)

A *type I error* (α) is the probability of rejecting the null hypothesis when it is true. A *type II error* (β) is the probability of failing to reject the null hypothesis when it is false. Power ($1-\beta$) is the probability of rejecting the null hypothesis when it is false, which is the goal.

A priori an acceptable level of significance (α) is specified, below which the null hypothesis is rejected. The null and alternative hypotheses are designed so that the type I error has the worse consequences, because this probability can be controlled.

The previous section on characteristics of frequency distributions described the relationship between the mean and the standard deviation. According to the empirical rule, 95% of the observations from a normally distributed data set will fall within 1.96 standard deviations from the mean. The *central limit theorem* also will help to explain how to make the jump from descriptive statistics to inferential statistics. It states that if random samples of n measurements are repeatedly drawn from a population with a finite mean μ and a standard deviation α, then when n is large, the relative frequency histogram for the sample means (calculated from the repeated samples) will be approximately normal with mean μ and standard deviation $\sigma/\sqrt{n}$.

Suppose many random samples each including 43 persons, are taken from the large population of persons who have hepatitis A, and the average incubation time period for each of the samples is recorded. If these means are presented on a histogram, the theoretical distribution of all the sample means would be approximately normally distributed, and the mean of this theoretical sampling distribution would approximate the mean in the entire population of hepatitis A cases in the large city. The standard deviation of this theoretical sampling distribution (i.e., *standard error*) of sample means would equal the standard deviation of the entire population divided by the square root of the sample size, or $\alpha/\sqrt{43}$. This result explains the theory behind statistical inference. In practice, only a single sample is selected for analysis and the results from that selected sample are compared with the theoretical distribution of all possible sample means from repeated samples from the population.

The theoretical sampling distribution from the hepatitis A example can be constructed assuming the null hypothesis is true. Under the null hypothesis, the mean in the population is 27 days; therefore, the mean of the sampling distribution of all possible samples containing 43 persons is 27 days. The standard deviation from the sample ($s = 3.7$ days) is used to estimate the population standard deviation (α). The standard deviation of the sampling distribution or the standard error (SE) approximated by $s/\sqrt{n}$) is $3.7/\sqrt{43} = 0.6$ (Fig. 2.3).

The further the sample mean lies from the hypothesized mean, the more likely the null hypothesis is to be false. In the actual sample, which includes 43 persons, the mean was 28.9 days. The probability can be calculated of observing a sample mean as extreme as $\bar{x} = 28.9$ days assuming that the sampling distribution of the mean is a normal distribution with a mean of 27 days and standard deviation of the mean of 0.6. The probability is 0.001. This probability is commonly referred to as the *p-value*. This value often is misinterpreted as the probability that the observed result was due to chance alone. The correct interpretation of a *p*-value,

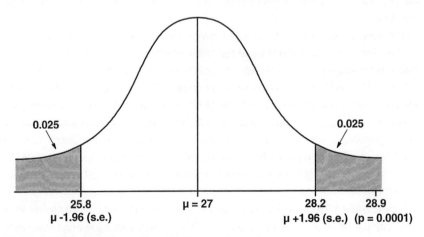

Figure 2.3. Theoretical sampling distribution of sample means.

which is a conditional probability, is the probability of obtaining a result from the sample as extreme or more extreme than the one observed given that the null hypothesis is true. In this example, it is unlikely ($p = 0.001$) that a sample mean of 28.9 would be observed given that the true mean incubation time period in the population was 27 days. This p-value is compared with a significance level (α), which is specified a priori. Suppose in this example $\alpha = 0.05$. Because the p-value is less than the specified significance level, the null hypothesis that $\mu = 27$ days is rejected, in favor of the alternate that the average incubation time period in the population is different from 27 days.

The confidence interval is based on the same theory as the significance test (e.g., the *central limit theorem*). The mean incubation time period for the 43 cases of hepatitis A is 28.9 days. That statistic is an estimate of the population parameter, or the average incubation time period in the population from which the sample came. Sampling error is associated with this estimate because of the variability in the selection of the sample. A statistic, such as "$\bar{x}$" is called a random variable. A confidence interval provides an interval within which the true average incubation time period in the population likely falls. A 95% confidence interval for the mean is calculated as $\bar{x} \pm 1.96 \cdot \text{SE}$. That value would differ for confidence intervals other than 95% or for nonnormally distributed data. For the hepatitis A data, the 95% confidence interval for the mean is constructed as $\bar{x} \pm 1.96 \cdot \text{SE} = 28.9 \pm 1.96 \cdot 0.6 = (27.7, 30.8)$.

The confidence interval provides 95% confidence that the true average incubation time period in the population falls between 27.7 and 30.8 days. Once a confidence interval is calculated, it either contains the true population parameter or it does not. If many samples of size 43 are selected, then of all the corresponding confidence intervals calculated, 95% of them will contain the true population parameter.

A relationship exists between the confidence interval and the test of significance. Some persons use the confidence interval as a method of significance testing. If the confidence interval does not contain the value of the parameter stated in the null hypothesis, then the null hypothesis is rejected.

Tests of significance for measures of association are based on related methods. For the typical 2×2 table that presents two levels of an exposure and two levels of outcome, the Fisher exact test can be performed to determine the exact probability (i.e., p-value) of observing a table as extreme or more extreme than the one observed, provided there is no association between exposure and disease. This test enumerates all possible 2×2 tables with the marginal totals fixed and sums the probability of those as extreme or more extreme than the one observed (Fleiss, 1982). When all of the expected values of the 2 x 2 table are above 5, using an approximate method is computationally easier. The theoretical distribution of a function of the observed and expected values is a *chi-square (χ^2) distribution*. A chi-square statistic is calculated from the data, and the probability of observing a chi-square as extreme or more extreme than the one observed can easily be determined under the null hypothesis of no association [see Fleiss (1982) for details on significance tests and confidence intervals for measures of association].

Modeling

Modeling is useful in assessing relationships in epidemiology. Deterministic models (e.g., decision analysis) are discussed in Chapter 6. Only *logistic regression* is described in this chapter. Logistic regression is a commonly used modeling technique in epidemiology.

A brief overview of stratified analysis may aid in understanding the need for and use of logistic regression. Often, when observing 2×2 tables and looking for associations between exposure and disease outcome, differences are suspected in these associations for various levels of a third variable. For example, one may suspect that the association between exposure and disease is different for males and females. The data can be stratified by gender and the appropriate measure of association can be observed for each stratum. Schlesselman (1982) and Fleiss (1982) provide details for analysis and significance testing of stratified data. Often, stratum-specific estimates differ from one another. For example, in males, the calculated measure of association may indicate a very strong relationship between exposure and disease, whereas in females, only a very weak association may exist. This relationship is called *effect modification* or *interaction*. Presentation of a single summary measure would be misleading; the stratum-specific results would be most accurate. Synergism is another concept related to interaction and effect modification that addresses the biological relationship between exposure and disease (Kleinbaum, 1993).

Another interrelationship among variables is *confounding*. Confounding is the process by which a relationship between disease and an exposure is distorted by the relationship of some third variable (i.e., the confounder) with the disease and the exposure of interest (Schlesselman, 1982). For a variable to be considered a confounder, it must be associated with the exposure of interest and with the disease outcome independent of the exposure. Age is often associated with disease and is therefore considered a potential confounder for many epidemiological studies. If the relationship between exposure and disease is similar for each of the age groups but different from the unstratified or crude measure of association (over all age groups combined), then evidence of confounding exists, and a summary measure that controls for the effect of the confounder (e.g., a Mantel-Haensel estimate) is necessary (Fleiss, 1982).

When conducting an epidemiological analysis, the basic 2×2 table analysis with stratified analysis should be used to assess potential confounders or effect modifiers. However, the data often become too sparse, particularly when stratifying among several variables. In this situation, logistic regression is most advantageous.

Frequently in epidemiological research, independent variables are evaluated to predict the dependent variable. This situation requires a *multivariable analysis*. The independent variables are the collection of the exposure(s) of interest, confounders, and/or effect modifiers. The dependent variable is a dichotomous variable (i.e., has only two possible values), which is usually whether or not a person becomes ill with the disease.

The logistic function, $f(y) = 1/(1 + e^{-y})$, often is used to model the probability of disease. As is true for all probabilities, $0 \leq f(y) \leq 1$. The conditional probability of disease (D) given the values of the independent variables $(x_1, \ldots, x_k)$, is modeled by the logistic model (Kleinbaum, Kupper, and Morgenstern, 1993):

$$p(D = 1 | x_1, x_2, x_3, \ldots, x_k) = 1 / 1 + e^{-(\alpha + \Sigma \beta_i x_i)}$$

Many statistical software packages provide maximum likelihood estimates for the βs and α in the above model. Once the βs and α are estimated, individual risks of disease can be calculated or compared. However, the individual risk can only be calculated for follow-up studies (Kleinbaum, 1994). In a case-control or cross-sectional study, the estimate has no meaning and therefore should not be used. The odds ratio is the most common statistic measured from logistic regression modeling (Kleinbaum 1994).

Software packages have facilitated the use of logistic regression in epidemiological analysis. The user must be aware of the complexity of this approach and evaluate the appropriateness of its use. The data (i.e., observing predictors, confounders, and effect modifiers) require a model building strategy [e.g., hierarchical backward elimination recommended by Kleinbaum (1994)]. Computer packages are unable to differentiate among the several types of variables. Logistic regression diagnostics (e.g., checking for collinearity among the variables) must also be employed (Kleinbaum, 1994).

Survival analysis is a second popular modeling procedure used in epidemiology. Survival analysis is used to model the time until an event (e.g., death). Besides the modeling techniques, there are several procedures designed to analyze such data. One such procedure is life-table analysis, which is a summary of the mortality experience of a population (Selvin, 1996). A complete description of life-table analysis and survival analysis is beyond the scope of this section. (Kleinbaum, 1996, Dawson-Saunders, 1994).

Attributable Risk

A measure of impact that has important implications in public health is *attributable risk* or (AR) attributable fraction. Attributable risk is defined by Lilienfeld (1994) as "the maximum proportion of a disease that can be attributed to a characteristic or etiological factor." If the exposure is a causal factor of the disease, the attributable risk provides a measure of what proportion of the disease can be attributed to the exposure. The remaining proportion equals the proportion of disease that would have occurred even in the absence of the exposure. The definition of attributable risk assumes that all other extraneous variables are distributed similarly among the exposed and nonexposed groups. In its simplest form, the formula for attributable risk is:

$$AR = \frac{\text{Risk (or rate) for exposed} - \text{Risk (or rate) for unexposed}}{\text{Risk (or rate) for exposed}}$$

See Kleinbaum et al (1993) for the AR formula that should be used when multiple risk factors are present.

In the incidence density example discussed earlier (Doll and Hill, 1964a,b), the rate for lung cancer deaths among smokers was 1.30 per 1000 person years. The rate for lung cancer deaths among nonsmokers was 0.07 per 1000 person-years. The attributable risk is calculated as $(1.30 - 0.07)/1.30 = 0.95$. Of all the lung cancer deaths, 95% can be attributed to smoking. If none of the persons in the population had ever smoked, 95% of all 133 deaths, or 126 of the deaths, would not have occurred as a result of lung cancer. The other seven deaths, however, would still be expected to occur.

Attributable risk is useful to help guide public health action. If a large proportion of the population becomes exposed to a particular risk factor that is strongly associated with a disease, this exposure should be eliminated or prevented whenever possible.

Forecasting

Forecasting is a method used to predict future events. *Mathematical models* are used to pattern data collected over time (often called *time-series* data). Once appropriate models are determined to fit existing observations, these models can be used to forecast future values for the series. Public health data are well suited for time-series models because they are so frequently collected over time.

There are two basic approaches to forecasting. A univariate approach that uses only the history of the series describes how the observations of a variable are related to past observations of the same variable. A multivariate approach accounts for external influences rather than simply past observations. A commonly used univariate approach for modeling time-series data is the Box-Jenkins methodology. Box-Jenkins methodology includes a large class of models. These models are also referred to as autoregressive moving average (ARIMA) models. The following is one example of an ARIMA model:

$$z_t = c + \phi_1 z_{t-1} + a_t$$

This defines the mathematical relationship between the current value of the variable z and its past values; c is a constant term, a_t is the probabilistic component, and ϕ_1 is the parameter to be estimated, which defines the relationship between z_t and z_{t-1} (Pankratz, 1983). This particular model is called an autoregressive model of order one, where the current value of the variable z_t is related to its immediate past value z_{t-1}. This model is only one of a family of models that can be explored. Once an appropriate model is selected to best represent a time series, diagnostic tests have been developed to determine the accuracy of the model and the forecasting ability (Pankratz, 1983). ARIMA models are particularly suited to series that demonstrate seasonality, which are frequently encountered in public health.

Once good models are developed to describe disease patterns, comparing actual results to those that were forecast can be critical for monitoring epidemics or simply changes in the disease process. This monitoring allows for quick public health response to changes in expected disease rates. Forecasting disease rates can be helpful not only for monitoring the behavior of disease patterns but also for disease prevention.

Summary and Conclusions

This chapter provides a general overview of important statistical methods for the analysis of public health data. A basic understanding of these methods is necessary to appropriately use and interpret the analysis of such data.

Statistics in public health is an evolving discipline. The scope of this chapter does not include all statistical topics. For example, in the section on modeling, only stochastic models, or probability-based models, are discussed. Researchers also utilize deterministic models, which do not reflect the role of chance in disease spread (Hethcote and Van Ark, 1992). Such deterministic models are often easier to analyze than the corresponding stochastic models. Several mathematical models are used for modeling HIV/AIDS (Hethcote and Van Ark, 1992).

Another evolving area in the field of statistics is *meta-analysis*. Hedges and Olkin (1985) state that "meta analysis is the rubric used to describe quantitative methods for combining evidence across studies." One of the steps required for making conclusions regarding causation is reproducibility of the results. The vast amount of information in the scientific literature and the increasing number of often related scientific studies have prompted the need for a scientific method that facilitates a summary of the results from several related studies. Typical epidemiological studies are aimed at summarizing data from all persons in a single study. A meta-analysis in aimed at synthesizing the summaries of data from persons in single studies across many studies (Hedges and Olkin, 1985).

Statistics in public health research will continue to develop. Software packages will continue to make it easier to perform appropriate analyses. It is important for such a scientific discipline to progress; however, it is equally important that the basic foundations for the methods be understood by its users.

References

Centers for Disease Control and Prevention. Comprehensive assessment of health needs two months after hurricane Andrew—Dade County, Florida, 1992. *MMWR Morb. Mortal. Wkly. Rep.* 42:434–437, 1993.

Cochran, W. G. *Sampling Techniques.* New York: W. H. Freeman & Co., 1977.

Daniel, W. W. *Biostatistics: Foundation for Analysis in the Health Sciences.* New York: John Wiley & Sons, 1995.

Dawson-Saunders, B., and Trapp, R. G. *Basic and Clinical Biostatistics.* Norwalk, CT: Appleton & Lange, 1994.

Dean, A. G., J. A. Dean, J. H. Burton, et al. A word processing, database, and statistics program for epidemiology on micro-computers. Epi Info, version 6. [Computer Program]. Atlanta, GA: Centers for Disease Control and Prevention, Public Health Service, U.S. Department of Health and Human Services, 1993.

Doll, R., and A. B. Hill. Mortality in relation to smoking: 10 years' observation of British doctors. *Br. Med. J.* 1:1399–1410, 1964a.

Doll, R., and A. B. Hill. Mortality in relation to smoking: 10 years' observation of British doctors. *Br. Med. J.* 1:1460–1467, 1964b.

Elandt-Johnson, R. C. Definition of rates: some remarks on their use and misuse. *Am. J. Epidemiol.* 102:267–271, 1975.

Fleiss, J. C. *Statistical Methods for Rates and Proportions.* New York: John Wiley & Sons, 1981.

Giri, N. C. *Introduction to Probability and Statistics.* New York: Marcel Dekker, Inc., 1993.

Gross, M. Oswego County revisited. *Public Health Rep.* 91:168–170, 1976.

Hedges, L. V., and I. Olkin. *Statistical Methods for Meta-analysis.* New York: Academic Press, Inc., 1985.

Hethcote, H. W., and J. W. Van Ark. *Lecture Notes in Biomathematics, Modeling HIV Transmission and AIDS in the United States.* New York: Springer-Verlag, 1992.

Kish, L. *Survey Sampling.* New York: John Wiley & Sons, 1965.

Kleinbaum, D. G., and L. L. Kupper, and H. Morgenstern. *Epidemiologic Research: Principles and Quantitative Methods.* Belmont, CA: Lifetime Learning Publications, 1993.

Kleinbaum, D. G. *Logistic Regression: A Self-Learning Text.* New York: Springer-Verlag, 1994.

Kleinbaum, D. G. *Survival Analysis: A Self-Learning Text.* New York: Springer-Verlag, 1996.

Lilienfeld, A. M. *Foundations of Epidemiology.* New York: Oxford University Press, 1994.

Moore, D. S., and G. P. McCabe. *Introduction to the Practice of Statistics.* New York: W. H. Freeman & Co., 1989.

Pankratz, A. *Forecasting with Univariate Box-Jenkins Models, Concepts and Cases.* New York: John Wiley & Sons, 1983.

Scheaffer, R. L., W. Mendenhall, and L. Ott. *Elementary Survey Sampling.* Boston, MA: Duxbury Press, 1986.

Schlesselman, J. J. *Case-Control Studies: Design, Conduct, Analysis*. New York: Oxford University Press, 1982.

Selvin, S. *Statistical Analysis of Epidemiologic Data*. New York: Oxford University Press, 1996.

Shah, B. V., B. G. Barnwell, P. N. Hunt, and L. M. LaVange. *SUDAAN user's manual*. Research Triangle Park, NC: Research Triangle Institute, 1991.

Williams, B. *Biostatistics: Concepts and Applications for Biologists*. New York: Chapman & Hall, 1993.

3

Data Sources for Public Health

STEPHEN B. THACKER
SCOTT F. WETTERHALL

> A single death is a tragedy. A million deaths is a statistic.
> —Joseph Stalin (1879–1953)

In public health, data are used for both research and program implementation. Sources of data can be categorized as vital statistics and census, registries, public health surveillance systems, surveys of populations or providers, epidemic investigations, research studies, and program evaluations. Data used in public health may be generated specifically for public health uses or may be obtained from sources that are collected for other purposes (e.g., workers' compensation or the Hazardous Materials Information Systems of the Department of Transportation). In this chapter, each of these types of data sources will be defined and illustrated. The strengths and weaknesses of each data source will be evaluated for specific uses. Applications of data to public health will be illustrated, and data issues of particular interest (e.g., confidentiality) will be discussed. Finally, new directions in data use in public health (e.g., informatics) and new data sources [e.g., managed care organizations (MCO)] will be addressed.

Data Sources

Vital Statistics and the Census

Mortality data most typically are derived from death certificates collected locally, collated at the state level, and analyzed at the national level by the National Center for Health Statistics (NCHS). All deaths and births in the United States are registered through this system, which provides a complete population enumera-

39

tion. At the local level, vital records systems are quite timely and have been used for surveillance of mortality associated with acute events (e.g., heat waves and influenza). However, national mortality data are not available for up to 3 years after the close of the calendar year (Kovar, 1989), although a 10% sample is available within 12 months.

Census data are collected every 10 years and updated in the interim. Such data provide the denominators for rate-based assessment of local and national data in public health.

Both vital records and census data are designed for complete enumeration. Although complete enumeration essentially occurs for vital records, because of U.S. burial laws, census data are limited by undercounting—particularly of special populations. These issues must be addressed before statistical tests are applied to the data.

Public Health Surveillance

Public health surveillance is the ongoing and systematic collection, analysis, and interpretation of outcome-specific data, closely integrated with the timely dissemination of those data to those responsible for preventing and controlling disease and injury (Thacker and Stroup, 1994). Surveillance data are collected from multiple sources, including many of the other data sources previously noted.

Traditional surveillance is illustrated by the National Notifiable Disease Surveillance System (Koo and Wetterhall, 1996). Physicians, laboratorians, and other health care providers are required by state law to report all cases of health conditions that are specified as being notifiable; most of these conditions are infectious in origin. Typically, a case report form is completed by a health care provider or laboratorian and mailed to the local or state health department. Authority to modify the list of notifiable diseases is often granted to the state health officer; in some states, each change must be newly legislated. Reporting is influenced by the disease severity, availability of public health measures, public concern, ease of reporting, and physician appreciation of public health practice in the community (Thacker and Stroup, 1994).

The Council of State and Territorial Epidemiologists determines which notifiable conditions should be reported from the state health department to the Centers for Disease Control and Prevention (CDC). The CDC also collaborates with state and local departments to establish specialized disease and injury reporting systems. Other federal agencies are involved in the collection of surveillance data. For example, the Food and Drug Administration (FDA) conducts postmarketing surveillance of adverse reaction to drugs (Faich et al., 1987), and the Consumer Product Safety Commission conducts surveillance on product-related injuries (Rivara et al., 1982).

Chronic disease investigators, however, typically combine data from vital statistics, population surveys, registries, and health services sources to assess the magnitude and changes in known risk factors, daily living habits, health care, major social and economic features, and morbidity and mortality (Thacker et al., 1995). The surveillance of risk factors for a condition is a particularly useful approach for chronic diseases both because of long latency between exposure and disease and the multifactorial etiology of many chronic conditions (Thacker et al., 1995).

Surveillance in environmental public health involves hazards and exposures as well as outcomes (see Table 3.1) (Thacker et al., 1996). Hazard surveillance focuses on trends in levels of hazards (e.g., chemical agents, physical agents, and biomechanical stressors), whereas exposure surveillance is the monitoring of the individual members of the population for the presence of an environmental agent or its clinically inapparent effects. An example of a hazard surveillance source is the environmental air monitoring data from 4000 state and local monitoring sites in the United States, which are mandated by the Clean Air Act. Data are collected and published routinely for six air pollutants covered by the national air quality standards (i.e., carbon monoxide, lead, nitrogen dioxide, ozone, particulate matter, and sulfur dioxide). Exposure surveillance is exemplified by the use of the results of blood lead testing among children (Pertowski, 1994). Such surveillance is used to assess the effectiveness of programs designed to reduce environmental lead hazards.

Public health agencies periodically obtain data from a sample of clinicians or institutions to monitor particular health events. For example, since the 1970s, the CDC has operated the National Nosocomial Infections Surveillance System, a national hospital laboratory-based system for the surveillance of hospital-acquired infections (Emori et al., 1991). At the local level, selected physicians often monitor the occurrence of acute disease trends. This type of system has been implemented on a national scale in France through its Minitel computer system and to a more limited degree in the United States and the Netherlands (Thacker and Stroup, 1994).

In a variation of this approach, the CDC's National Institute of Occupational Safety and Health has maintained a sentinel health event verification system for occupational risk, which is a state-based network of health care providers that focuses on reporting specific occupational conditions (Baker, 1989).

Surveillance data vary in their quality and often are incomplete and unrepresentative. Depending on their intended use, they may vary in sensitivity and specificity. For example, systems used to detect acute outbreaks of severe diseases may be designed to be sensitive and often pick up conditions that are false-positive. Other systems (usually these are used for archival purposes) yield more specific data but often are not timely.

Various forms of regression analyses (and more recently, time-series analyses) have been applied successfully to surveillance data both to monitor trends and to forecast future trends in disease and injury occurrence. Sentinel surveillance data

TABLE 3.1.   Selected National Data Sources that Support Environmental Public Health Surveillance, United States*

Title[†]	Category[‡]	Scope	Responsible Organizations	Sources of Data
Aerometric Informational Retrieval	H	National	Environmental Protection Agency	Air monitoring sites
Ambulatory Sentinel Practice Network for North America	O	National**	Ambulatory Sentinel Practice Network Network	Family physicians
Drug Abuse Warning Network	E,O	National	National Institute on Drug Abuse	Emergency rooms, medical examiners/coroners
Hazardous Substances Emergency Events Surveillance System	H,O	Five states	Agency for Toxic Substances and Disease Registry (ATSDR)	State agencies, hospitals, fire/ police departments
Hazardous Materials Information System	H,O	National	Department of Transportation	Highway patrol
Medical Examiner/Coroner Information Sharing System	E,O	National**	Centers for Disease Control and Prevention (CDC)	Medical examiners/ coroners
Medicare Provider Analysis and Review	O	National	Health Care Financing Administration	Office-based medical practices, hospital discharge data
McAuto	O	National**	McDonnel-Douglas Corporation	Hospital discharge abstracts
National Ambulatory Medical Care Survey	O	National	National Center for Health Statistics (CDC)	Ambulatory-care providers
National Disease and Therapeutic Index	E,O	National	IMS, Inc.	Office-based medical practices
National Exposure Registry	H,E	National	Agency for Toxic Substances and Disease Registry (ATSDR)	Personal interviews

System	Category‡	Scope	Source	Data
National Health Assessment and Nutrition Examination Survey	E,O	National	National Center for Health Statistics (CDC)	Population survey respondents
National Health Interview Survey	H,O	National	National Center for Health Statistics (CDC)	Household interview respondents
National Hospital Discharge Survey	O	National	National Center for Health Statistics (CDC)	Hospital discharge abstracts
Professional Activities Study	O	National	Commission of Professional and Hospital Activities	Hospital discharge abstracts
Surveillance, Epidemiology, and End-Results (SEER) Program	O	National**	National Cancer Institute, National Institutes of Health	Cancer registry
Toxic Release Inventory	H	National	Environmental Protection Agency	Industry
Vital records	O	National	National Center for Health Statistics (CDC), States	Death certificates, birth certificates
Water Data Storage and Retrieval System	H	National	Department of the Interior, U.S. Geological Survey	Multiple soil and water sites

*References available on request.

†References to these systems available from authors on request.

‡Category: H = hazard, E = exposure, O = outcome.

**Includes selected states or localities only.

are most typically convenience samples, and therefore statistical testing has limited application. When statistical tests are used, the nature of the sample must be accounted for. Often, particularly with noninfectious diseases, data sources collected for other reasons are used for surveillance. Investigators must take particular care when applying statistical tools to such data sources, since they may have been collected using complex designs.

Surveys

Surveys are systemic investigations conducted on a population. The CDC's NCHS is responsible for several national surveys that monitor the nation's health (Kovar, 1989). The National Health Interview Survey is an ongoing survey of 40,000 households. This survey uses a multistage probability sample of the civilian, non-institutionalized population of the United States. In 1981, the CDC's Behavioral Risk Factor Surveillance System (BRFSS) enabled state health departments to use random telephone dialing for recurrent, cross-sectional, state-wide surveys of risk factor information (Siegel et al., 1991). State health departments have used information from this system to support personal risk reduction and disease prevention activities (e.g., the New Hampshire Indoor Smoking Act) (CDC, 1990). Health jurisdictions at all levels of government conduct surveys of specific populations (e.g., workers, schoolchildren, and populations at risk during epidemics) to obtain information critical for public health practice (Gregg et al., 1996).

Surveys also can be conducted of institutions or their populations. For example, the National Hospital Discharge Survey of NCHS is a continuing nationwide sample survey of short-stay U.S. hospitals that has been conducted since 1965 (Kovar, 1989). Regional- and state-based hospital discharge systems also have been used for surveillance. The National Health Assessment and Nutritional Examination Survey is conducted periodically on a nationally representative sample of the population by NCHS and combines information from personal interviews with physical examination and laboratory data. The NCHS's National Ambulatory Medical Care Survey and the privately financed National Disease and Therapeutic Index provide data concerning diagnosis and drug therapy from physician practices throughout the United States.

Surveys may be conducted as simple random, systematic samples, or (as with the National Health Interview Survey) they may involve complex design. The nature of the design of the survey defines the appropriate statistical tools used to analyze data collected. Sometimes (as with BRFSS surveys, where data are combined from multiple states to make national estimates) complex statistical challenges arise.

Registries

Population-based registries are established to obtain information on all cases of a health event. Typically, registries are established by researchers to identify cases through several sources (e.g., schools, hospitals, and laboratories) and are not linked to public health prevention and control activities. Registries require extensive confirmation of cases leading to longer lag times between of the health event and the reporting of such events. The Surveillance, Epidemiology, and End Results (SEER) program of the National Cancer Institute covers about 10% of the U.S. population (Gloeckler-Ries et al., 1990). The program provides data that are used to monitor long-term trends of cancer incidence and mortality, assess cancer trends, and develop priorities for allocating resources for cancer research and control. Currently, approximately 30 states have population-based registries. The Medicare data system compiled by the Health Care Financing Administration covers hospitalization expenses for about 95% of the elderly population and can be used as a registry for some serious illnesses among the elderly (Health Care Financing Administration, 1989).

Registries are designed for complete enumeration of persons with particular diseases or exposures. However, registries may be limited by both underregistration and selection bias. Statistical testing must account for these factors.

Epidemic Investigations

One of the most widely recognized activities in public health practice is the investigation of epidemics (Gregg et al., 1996). These investigations are usually done at the state and local levels and are sometimes triggered by surveillance data. However, nationally recognized investigations (e.g., those of the epidemics of legionnaires' disease and toxic-shock syndrome) are most visible to the general public. In such investigations, data are first collected to describe the nature and extent of the problems. The problems are redefined; hypotheses are generated and then tested, usually through analytic methods (e.g., a case-control study). Surveillance systems are often set up to collect new cases, and provisional case definitions are established both for surveillance and for analytic studies (Swygert et al., 1990). In the case of a prolonged epidemic, additional studies may be built on the results of the initial analysis, and long-term surveillance activities may be established. Occasionally, multisite outbreaks (including multistate outbreaks) lead to collaborative investigations on a regional or national scale.

Epidemic studies often include various study designs (e.g., case-control studies and cohort studies) and frequently investigators establish surveillance systems for the course of the epidemic. Statistical tests appropriate for the particular study design in an investigation must be used.

Research

An essential data source for public health practice is population-based research. Analytic research ranging from descriptive studies to case-control studies, cohort studies, and randomized, controlled clinical trials form an important scientific underpinning of good public health practice. Such research is undertaken in academia, industry, and other segments of the private sector, as well as all levels of government.

Research studies range from randomized, controlled clinical trials to cohort and case-control studies. Each of these study designs generates extensive methodological considerations and is addressed in separate publications.

Program Evaluations

An essential part of public health practice is an evaluation of intervention programs. These evaluations may include an assessment of process (e.g., number of immunizations given) and/or an outcome (e.g., number of cases of measles). Different methodological designs are used to evaluate programs, depending on the size and duration of such programs and the number of persons affected. Often program evaluations will use data from research studies and surveillance systems to assess the impact of programs. In addition, economic methods (e.g., cost-effectiveness analyses) are used as part of the overall assessment of prevention activities.

Alternative Data Sources

Whereas public health practitioners often collect data for specific public health uses, data systems maintained by sources as diverse as the National Highway Traffic Safety Administration, the Department of Transportation, the Department of Justice, and FDA also have been used for public health purposes. An example of such a data system is the Hazardous Materials Information System of the Department of Transportation, which was established in 1971. The system provides reporting of spills associated with interstate commerce on a voluntary basis (U.S. Congress, Office of Technology Assessment, 1986). Such data, while incomplete, complement other activities at the state and local levels to monitor environmental hazard risks. Such systems often are the only available source of information for particular issues of public health importance. These systems, however, often are not integrated at the state and national levels of public health surveillance and prevention activities. Nonetheless, despite this lack of coordination and specificity, such systems have proven useful in the development and assessment of public health programs.

Medical records are gaining increasing recognition for potential use in the field of public health. At the national level, Medicare data have been adapted for research purposes; locally and regionally, managed care organizations have established research activities based on their patient populations (Health Care Financing Administration, 1989).

Uses of Public Health Data: Case Studies

A comprehensive public health surveillance and information system has been described as a network of compatible health information systems linked electronically that is readily accessible to public health practitioners on a timely basis (Thacker and Stroup, 1994). In addition to public health officials, private laboratories, clinics, schools, and other private sector organizations would have access to such data. Such a distributed data system also would include health information from research and other alternative data sources. Those who maintain the system would have to address concerns of common data elements, timeliness, accessibility, confidentiality, and flexibility. An appropriate computer system would need to be developed based on experience with national computer systems in the United States, France, and other countries.

Data from such surveillance systems have many uses. One scheme describes immediate, annual, and archival types of uses for surveillance data (Thacker and Stroup, 1994). Data from other health information systems, whether collected primarily for public health or other reasons, would have similar uses, although for the most part, not for immediate use in epidemic detection and control. In terms of each of these uses, the various data systems have relative strengths and weaknesses. The examples described in the following paragraphs will illustrate the challenges met by public health practitioners in balancing the strengths and weaknesses when addressing particular health problems.

Monitoring the Health of a Community/Population: Cardiovascular Disease

Recognizing that cardiovascular disease is the leading cause of death in the United States, a state health officer needs information on the prevalence of certain risk factors for this disease that can be used to compare his or her state's experience with national trends and to identify subgroups within his or her jurisdiction that may be at higher risk.

The BRFSS, which collects information on smoking, sedentary lifestyle, obesity, hypertension, and diabetes, is well suited for obtaining this type of information (Siegel et al., 1991). BRFSS telephone surveys can result in data from a sample that is representative of the entire state. In addition, results are timely, becoming available usually within about 6 months of collection. However, the system also has limitations. Because the system uses telephone interviews, the collected information is self-reported, which may lead to inaccuracies, particularly for weight, presence of diabetes, or degree of exercise. Because the system is designed to provide statewide estimates using samples averaging 1500 respondents, the data cannot be disaggregated to provide estimates for smaller units; for example, counties (even though these would be the most valuable estimates for the county health officials). The system can be modified, but adding new questions can be time consuming and expensive because of the need for pilot testing, modifying the interview protocol, and training.

Other sources of data can be used to obtain information on behavioral risk factors, but with less efficiency or greater cost. Surveys—particularly those with health examinations—can be designed to obtain accurate information even in smaller geographic units, but this approach is costly and time consuming, particularly if anticipated as ongoing monitoring. Any gain in precision and accuracy must be weighed against these additional costs. Vital records (e.g., death certificates) contain information on some risk factors (e.g., smoking and diabetes). However, (*1*) this data source can be less helpful in monitoring the health of the population because the completeness of reporting varies by practitioner, (*2*) information is not collected on all of the risk factors of interest, and (*3*) there are delays in obtaining these data. A registry of persons who have been diagnosed with some other form of ischemic heart disease might exist. Detailed information on risk factors would be available, but their representativeness to the general population would be severely limited. Sentinel surveillance systems would not be particularly useful in capturing information on risk factors in the general population because data are incomplete and biased. Research studies, especially longitudinal studies of cohorts or communities (e.g., the Framingham Study) have provided valuable information about the interplay of risk factors and the natural history of cardiovascular disease, but their considerable expense and limited generalizability impedes their usefulness in tracking populations over time. Thus, a system based on ongoing telephone surveys to collect information about self-reported behaviors represents the preferred choice for monitoring the health of the surveyed community over time.

Advocating for Health: Breast Cancer

The governor of a small industrialized state announces that there will be a 10% increase in his next year's budget for health and social services. These increases, amounting to several million dollars, will be used to fund a comprehensive cancer control plan. Under this plan, the state department of health will identify the localities with the highest prevalence of certain cancers, evaluate the occurrence of behavior and environmental risk factors for cancer, and develop several new screening and prevention programs. The state will purchase a mobile mammography laboratory to provide screening examinations to residents of inner city neighborhoods. The governor developed this plan in response to a national report that indicating that his state has the highest number of deaths from breast cancer, and that many of these deaths could be prevented through early screening. The governor is concerned that persons will learn of the state's ranking and question whether the state has an unhealthy environment created by pollution from the many chemical and automotive industries located there.

The national report, in addition to ranking states by mortality rate, reported that the population attributable risk (PAR) for nonutilization of mammography was 19.3%. The PAR is commonly interpreted as the proportion of disease or death in a population that is attributable to a particular risk factor (Hahn et al., 1990). Calculation of the PAR requires both (*1*) an estimate of the prevalence of the risk factor in the population and (*2*) a measure of the strength of association (i.e., an odds ratio or risk ratio) between the risk factor and the adverse health outcome. In this instance, the National Health Interview Survey data were used to estimate the prevalence of nonutilization of mammography, and the relative risk was determined from a randomized clinical trial conducted as early as the 1960s.

Population attributable risks have appeal in advocating for health because they provide a simple and understandable summary measure. Making the data understandable is the first step in presenting data to legislators and others who control resources (Sederburg, 1992). The inviting logic is to conclude that screening all women will prevent nearly one-fifth of all deaths caused by breast cancer. Nonetheless, those who use PARs for advocacy purposes must understand their limitations. The measure of association may be derived from studies of groups who bear little resemblance to the current population of interest. The risk estimates may have been calculated without accounting for the affect of potential confounding factors (e.g., family history of breast cancer). In addition, risk factors may interact with one another (i.e., the presence of one risk factor may increase or decrease the effect of another risk factor). Rarely do health officials have precise knowledge of the joint prevalence and independent effects of multiple risk factors on the health outcome of interest. Thus, PARs can be viewed as approximate measures at best.

Evaluating Program Outcome: Teen Pregnancy

Reducing the number of pregnancies among adolescent girls is a national objective that has been adopted as a health promotion goal by many state health agencies. In one state, during the previous legislative session, the assembly authorized use of funds by the state health officer to develop outreach programs (e.g., educational programs) for high-risk groups to achieve these goals. Because this topic is contentious and politically volatile, the legislators want to be briefed on the current impact of these programs before additional funding is provided.

Demonstrating a decline in the rate of pregnancy among adolescents after the prevention programs have been implemented should favorably influence the legislators. Documenting changes in this rate requires accessing and analyzing four different types of data: the size of the population, the number of live births, number of abortions, and level of sexual activity (Wilson, 1994).

The decennial census provides authoritative counts on the size of the population of interest. Comparison of yearly changes in rates may require use of intercensal estimates, which introduce some uncertainty into the calculation of rates. The vital registration system provides virtually complete data on the number of births in the United States. Since 1989, the U.S. Standard Certificate of Live Birth, which states use as a model for developing their own certificates, has included new items on medical and behavioral factors that can be used to characterize more fully adolescents and others in high-risk pregnancy groups. More recently, several states have begun using electronic birth certificates to accelerate the registration process. Despite these enhancements, data concerning births may not become available for use at the state level until 18 months after a given calendar year.

Currently, 45 central health agencies collect information on the number of legal induced abortions, but previous studies have shown that these counts underestimate (by about 11%) the number of abortions obtained by the Alan Guttmacher Institute, which obtains information directly from abortion providers (Koonin et al., 1996). In addition, some states do not collect information concerning the age or the state of residence of the person obtaining the abortion.

To obtain information concerning sexual activity, many states have begun periodic administration of the school-based Youth Risk Behavior Survey, a multistage sampling survey of high school students (Kann et al., 1996). To improve comparability across sites, CDC, with its partners, developed a core questionnaire and now provides ongoing technical assistance in planning surveys and analyzing data.

Quantifying temporal changes in rates of adolescent pregnancy raises several issues. First, information must be obtained and consolidated from different data sources. Delays in obtaining data may decrease the usefulness in attempting to show program impact and justify expenditures. Underreporting the number of abortions may underestimate the rate of adolescent pregnancy. Not having information on the state of residence of the person obtaining the abortion can further complicate interpretation, particularly in jurisdictions (e.g., New York and Washington, DC) where the availability of abortion services may differ from that in contiguous areas. The difficulty in using surveys to measure accurately certain sensitive behaviors (e.g., sexual activity) is well known. Survey coverage may not include certain high-risk groups—the Youth Behavioral Factor Risk Survey misses adolescents who are no longer attending school. Finally, within the broader context of preventing adolescent pregnancy, the intent of the program services that are being evaluated may influence the analysis of the data. If the intent of the program is to reduce the proportion of adolescents of a certain age who have engaged in sexual intercourse, then the population at risk will be comprised of adolescents. Alternatively, if the intent is to evaluate the impact of family planning services, then pregnancy rates should be calculated using the sexually experienced adolescent population rather than the entire adolescent population. Thus, the purpose of the evaluation needs to be explicitly stated.

Evaluating Programs: Influenza

Each year, influenza continues to cause significant morbidity and mortality in the United States, particularly among the elderly and persons with certain underlying chronic diseases. Effective vaccines are available, but because the influenza virus can undergo rapid antigenic change, each year public health officials must select the vaccine subcomponents and commercial manufacturers must produce and distribute the vaccine before influenza season begins. Evaluating influenza prevention and control efforts is a complex process that requires collecting and synthesizing information from multiple data sources in a timely manner (Brammer et al., 1997). In addition to having measures of disease impact, public health officials need to have information regarding vaccine coverage (particularly in high-risk groups) and laboratory data that characterize which viruses are predominant.

Measures of disease impact derive from five sources: reports from state epidemiologists, a sentinel physician network, a mortality reporting system, investigation of outbreaks, and laboratory results. Each week, state and territorial epidemiologists report the level of influenza activity in their jurisdictions as widespread, regional, sporadic, or absent. This system provides a rapid, qualitative overview of influenza activity in each of the states. Sources used to make these assessments include notifiable disease data, reports from local health officers, viral isolates from local and state public laboratories, reports of influenza-like outbreaks, and the media. Although each level of influenza activity has been defined (e.g., "widespread" connotes either outbreaks of influenza-like illness or culture-confirmed influenza in counties comprising ≥50% of the state's population), in practice a considerable variability may exist across states in how these definitions are applied.

A group of 140 volunteer family-practice physicians participate in a sentinel surveillance network by reporting (from October through May) the number of patient visits, the number of patients with influenza-like illness (ILI), and the number of hospitalizations for patients with ILI, by age group. In an attempt to standardize reporting practices, ILI is defined as an illness characterized by fever of 100°F or greater and cough or sore throat in the absence of some other confirmed diagnosis. Such a case definition is sensitive but not particularly specific. This sentinel system is a simple, easy-to-operate system that provides timely data. The system is a useful adjunct to the other components of influenza surveillance—one that provides a window into the medical practices of a limited number of primary-care providers, although the representativeness and the generalizability of the data from this system are difficult to assess.

Each Friday, vital registrars in 122 U.S. cities report the number of death certificates for which pneumonia was an underlying cause or influenza a contributory cause of death. With historical data used to construct a pneumonia and influenza baseline curve, this system can rapidly identify periods when an "excess" number of deaths is occurring. Unlike the routine system of reporting vital statistics (for which there may be 2-year delays in obtaining data), results from the system are published each week in *Morbidity and Mortality Weekly Report.* Thus, this system is simple and extremely timely. The system has not proven to be particularly flexible; however, with few resources supporting this voluntary system, attempts to modify the system to capture data concerning deaths resulting from other causes has met minimal success.

State health departments, occasionally with assistance from CDC, often investigate outbreaks of febrile illness, which may occur in schools, nursing homes, and other chronic care facilities. When influenza outbreaks occur in certain self-contained populations (e.g., nursing homes) where the residents have medical or age-related indications for receiving annual influenza vaccines (as well as records documenting receipt of vaccination), these outbreak investigations can provide valuable information about vaccine efficacy.

Each week, 70 World Health Organization collaborating laboratories report the number of specimens received for testing respiratory viruses and the number of specimens that test positive for certain influenza antigenic strains. State and local health department laboratories comprise the majority of collaborating laboratories. Although the collection of specimens is not done systematically (i.e., on the basis of some sampling system), but rather reflects submissions by clinical providers, data from this laboratory system have accurately characterized the circulating strains of virus and are used to formulate the composition for the subsequent year's recommended vaccine.

Monitoring vaccine coverage for influenza poses several challenges. Under ideal circumstances, health officials would like to know the vaccine coverage within each targeted risk group. Although manufacturing and vaccine distribution data may be available, such information has not been useful in estimating coverage. Currently, surveys (e.g., the National Health Interview Survey of BRFSS) provide the simplest method of obtaining information, but these surveys suffer from lack of timeliness. Results may take from 6 months to a year to be reported—a brief interval for many conditions, but not particularly helpful to health officials who, if faced with an alarming increase in deaths, must consider lack of vaccine efficacy versus insufficient coverage as possible explanations. New sources of data (e.g., administrative billing systems) hold promise for monitoring vaccine coverage, but methods for routinely collecting and using these data have not been established.

Privacy and Confidentiality

Anyone who collects, transfers, distributes, provides upon request, or analyzes public health data should be familiar with the concepts of *privacy* and *confidentiality*. These are rapidly evolving issues that reflect the complex interplay of personal rights, ethical concerns, legal responsibility, and societal interest in general welfare and public health. Privacy, aptly described as a "deeply felt but elusive concept," has been defined in the legal sense as the "right to be let alone" (Lowrance, 1997). The construct reflects the notion of what personally identifiable information should be permitted to be collected and stored. Confidentiality reflects the responsibility on the part of those who hold or have access to personally identifiable data not to divulge it to others in a manner or degree that is inconsistent with the understanding of original disclosure under which the data were originally collected. Personally identifiable data are those that can be used directly (e.g., personal name), via linkage (e.g., social security number), or by deduction (e.g., a group of demographic or other distinguishing characteristics) to identify an individual.

Fundamental changes in the delivery and payment of personal health services and the practice of public health have focused interest on issues of privacy and confidentiality. These changes are underway within a context of rapidly evolving technology that permits compiling, storing, and sharing large amounts of sensitive health information. The growth of managed care has placed the medical care (and medical records) of sizable numbers of persons under the responsibility of large, for-profit organizations. Payment of health services requires transfer of electronic data, including diagnostic information, among service providers and payors. The mosaic of computer systems and networks fosters an interconnectivity that can permit linking of medical data with social, financial, and even legal information. Research in molecular biology advances our knowledge of the genetic basis of disease and offers methods for identifying persons at increased risk for certain health outcomes. In the wrong hands, however, this same information may be used to withhold employment or to deny life insurance. Thus, in the absence of necessary safeguards, these electronic data can provide composite information that can be used to manipulate and harm individuals.

Unfortunately, current protections are largely based on a patchwork of laws and regulations that date back to the preelectronic age (Gostin, 1995). Currently, no single federal statute protects the confidentiality of all personally identifiable data. The Privacy Act of 1974 prohibits certain disclosures of information without written consent of the individual, but many exceptions to this practice are permitted under the aegis of "routine uses" (Gostin, 1995).

Moreover, the Privacy Act generally does not pertain to health information not collected by the federal government. The Freedom of Information Act of 1966, enacted to permit the public to gain greater access to collected information, nonetheless contains several exemptions that have been invoked by federal agencies to avoid disclosure of personal information. Federally funded research involving human subjects, which falls under the "Federal Policy for the Protection of Human Subjects," requires review by an Institutional Review Board, with approval contingent on the assurance that provisions for protecting the privacy and confidentiality of the subjects are enacted. Confidentiality assurances that protect against disclosure, even under subpoena or court order, can be granted under provisions of the Public Health Service Act, but these assurances rarely are granted, and only for extremely sensitive data (e.g., information concerning illegal drug use). State privacy legislation varies widely in the degree of restrictiveness, granting of authority for access to data, and even the conditions and diseases covered by privacy and confidentiality protections.

Several recent developments will influence this complex mosaic of principles, practices, laws, and regulations. The federal Health Insurance Portability and Accountability Act of 1996 has provisions that will encourage sharing data (by establishing standards for electronic data interchange) as well as protect the privacy of individually identifiable health information (through either legislation or regulation). Several federal privacy bills have been introduced during the past few legislative sessions (Lowrance, 1997). In general, these bills attempt to establish uniform national rules for collecting, protecting, and disclosing personally identifiable health data.

In concert with establishing a consistent legal framework for addressing issues of privacy and confidentiality, technical practices and procedures are evolving rapidly to ensure the security of electronic health information. Security represents the measures used by individuals and organizations to protect the confidentiality of data. Recommended procedures include authentication of users, limiting access to a need-to-know basis, audit trails, physical security, controlling external access, and ongoing testing of security measures. The training and sensitizing of workers who handle personally identifiable data is critical in the success of any security system. Regardless of what system of procedures and controls is established, however, public health officials acknowledge the need for balance between providing access and protecting privacy and confidentiality. Striking the proper balance between these two demands will require continued discussion and debate within an arena of rapidly evolving issues.

New Directions

The recent developments that have focused attention on issues of privacy and confidentiality—new forms of health service delivery and new ways of practicing public health in an era of rapid technological change—will also influence the creation of future sources of data in public health. *Public health informatics* has been broadly defined as the use of information technology in the practice of public health. Advances in public health informatics will create innovative methods for accessing new sources and types of data.

The information systems of an MCO are examples of new sources of data that may be used for public health purposes. Currently, more than 70 million Americans receive health care through an arrangement with an MCO. With enrollment of its members, MCOs provide longitudinal care (often including preventive services) for a defined population. Thus, these circumstances permit ongoing assessment of effectiveness of medical practices. Data from MCOs have been used to monitor vaccine recipients for adverse reactions (Chen et al., 1997). The feasibility of conducting public health surveillance through MCOs is being evaluated.

Despite these promising features, using data from MCOs poses several challenges. The existing systems, which generally were established for administrative purposes, may not record outcome data (i.e., health events). Second, MCOs range in structure from group staff models (in which a single information system connects all practitioners) to an individual practice association (IPA)—a group of providers who have agreed to treat patients under specified terms arranged with the payor. With IPAs, therefore, the "information system" may be a conglomeration of separate, nonintegrated systems that are difficult to access. Finally, many plans currently experience a large degree of turnover in membership. Without a universal patient identifier available, tracking patients from plan to plan is not possible.

Electronic birth registration exemplifies a new type of data. Presently, hospitals may submit electronic data to vital registrars for recording births. Electronic birth data may be the first entry into a future computer-based patient record (Dick et al., 1991). Such a record may contain the entire health history of an individual. With access to such an electronic system of records, public health officials and others with legitimate needs will be able to monitor the health of the population on an ongoing basis. Before computer-based patient records find widespread use, however, issues such as implementing a unique health identifier, ensuring adequate safeguards for security and confidentiality, and adopting standards (e.g., for defining and coding variables and for telecommunications) need to be resolved.

Mechanisms for accessing data will continue to improve. Currently, many data sets exist on individual computers (with limited access) or as public use data tapes (e.g., vital records or the National Hospital Discharge Survey). Use of such data requires analyzing with and obtaining appropriate software and other tools. More recently, with the growth of the Internet, many state health departments provide access to tabular data via their World Wide Web pages. Providing even greater flexibility, CDC WONDER is an Internet-based system that permits the user to access more than 40 databases with specific queries. For example, the user can request public health surveillance data regarding AIDS for specified years, or examine the leading causes of death within a specific county.

CDC WONDER reflects many of the important trends influencing future access to public health data (Friede et al., 1994). The future will include widespread connectivity (via the Internet or its successor), enhanced database storage, rapid indexing of records, and powerful "search engines" for submitting and retrieving queries. Untested but envisioned is the creation of health "data warehouses" comprising computer-based patient records where data mining [i.e., using statistical rules to identify patterns (e.g., disease outbreaks)] is commonly performed. Regardless of which technologies are developed, their purpose will continue to enhance the access and use of data to protect and improve the health of the public.

References

Baker, E. L. Sentinel event notification system for occupational risks (SENSOR): the concept. *Am. J. Public Health* 79(Suppl.):18–20, 1989.

Brammer, L., K. Fukuda, N. Arden, et al. Influenza surveillance—United States, 1992–93 and 1993–94. In: CDC Surveillance Summaries, January 31, 1997. *MMWR Morb. Mortal. Wkly. Rep.* 46(No. SS-1):1–28, 1997.

Centers for Disease Control. State coalition for prevention and control of tobacco use. *MMWR Morb. Mortal. Wkly. Rep.* 39:476–485, 1990.

Chen, R. T., J. W. Glasser, P. H. Rhodes, et al. The Vaccine Safety Datalink Project: A New Tool for Improving Vaccine Safety Monitoring in the United States. *Pediatrics* 99:765–773, 1997.

Dick, R. S., E. B. Steen, (Eds.). *The Computer-Based Patient Record: An Essential Technology for Health Care*. Revised edition. Committee on Improving the Patient Record, Institute of Medicine. Washington, DC: National Academy Press, 1991.

Emori, T. G., D. H. Culver, T. C. Horan, et al. National Nosocomial Infections Surveillance systems (NNISS): description of surveillance methods. *Am. J. Infect. Control* 19:19–35, 1991.

Faich, G. A., D. Knapp, M. Dreis, et al. National adverse drug reaction surveillance—1985. *JAMA* 257:2068–2070, 1987.

Friede, A., D. H. Rosen, and J. A. Reid. CDC WONDER: a cooperative processing architecture for public health. *J. Am. Med. Informatics Assoc.* 1:303–312, 1994.

Gloeckler-Ries, L. A., B. F. Hankey, and B. K. Edwards, (Eds). *Cancer Statistics Review. 1973–1987.* Bethesda, MD: National Cancer Institute, NIH Publication No. 90–2789, 1990.

Gostin, L. O. Health information privacy. *Cornell Law Rev.* 80:451–528, 1995.

Gregg, M. B., R. C. Dicker, and R. A. Goodman. *Field Epidemiology.* New York: Oxford University Press, 1996.

Hahn, R. A., S. M. Teutsch, R. B. Rothenberg. Chronic disease reports from the MMWR Vol. 38 (1989) and Vol. 39 (1990). MMWR Compilation, October 12, 1–9, 1990.

Health Care Financing Administration. *Medicare Enrollment, 1986–87.* Baltimore: U.S. Department of Health and Human Services, Health Care Financing Administration, HCFA Publication No. 03282, 1989.

Kann, L., C. W. Warren, J. L. Collins, et al. Youth risk behavior surveillance—United States, 1995. In: CDC Surveillance Summaries, September 27, 1996. *MMWR Morb. Mortal. Wkly. Rep.* 45(No. SS-4): 1–83, 1996.

Koo, D., and S. F. Wetterhall. History and current status of the National Notifiable Diseases Surveillance System. *J. Public Health Management Pract.* 2:4–10, 1996.

Koonin, L. M., J. C. Smith, M. Ramick, and C. A. Green. Abortion surveillance—United States, 1992. In: CDC Surveillance Summaries, May 3, 1996. *MMWR Morb. Mortal. Wkly. Rep.* 45(No. SS-3):1–36, 1996.

Kovar, M. G. *Data systems of the National Center for Health Statistics.* Hyattsville, MD: National Center for Health Statistics, Centers for Disease Control, (Vital and health statistics, Series 1. DHHS Publication No. (PHS)89–1325, 1989.

Lowrance, W. W. *Privacy and Health Research: A Report to the U.S. Secretary of Health and Human Services.* U. S. Department of Health and Human Services, 1997, pp. 1–81.

Pertowski, C. A. Lead poisoning. In: *From Data to Action: CDC's Public Health Surveillance for Women, Infants, and Children,* edited by L. S. Wilcox, and J. S. Marks. Atlanta, GA: Centers for Disease Control and Prevention, 1994, pp. 311–319.

Rivara, F. P., A. B. Bergman, J. P. Lo Gerfo, et al. Epidemiology of childhood injuries: II. Sex differences in injury rates. *Am. J. Dis. Child.* 136:502–506, 1982.

Sederburg, W. A. Perspectives of the legislator: allocating resources. In: *Proceedings of the 1992 International Symposium on Public Health Surveillance,* edited by S. F. Wetterhall. *MMWR Morb. Mortal. Wkly. Rep.* 41(Suppl.):37–48, 1992.

Siegel, P. Z., R. M. Brackbill, E. L. Frazier, et al. Behavioral risk factor surveillance, 1986–1990. *MMWR Morb. Mortal. Wkly. Rep.* 40(No.SS-4):1–23, 1991.

Swygert, L. A., E. F. Maes, L. E. Sewell, et al. Eosinophilia-myalgia syndrome: results of national surveillance. *JAMA* 264:1698–1703, 1990.

Thacker, S. B., and D. F. Stroup. Future directions for comprehensive public health surveillance and health information systems in the United States. *Am. J. Epidemiol.* 140: 383–397, 1994.

Thacker, S. B., D. F. Stroup, R. G. Parrish, et al. Surveillance in environmental public health: issues, systems, and sources. *Am. J. Public Health* 86:633–638, 1996.

Thacker, S. B., D. F. Stroup, R. B. Rothenberg, et al. Public health surveillance for chronic conditions: a scientific basis for decisions. *Stat. Med.* 14:629–641, 1995.

U. S. Congress, Office of Technology Assessment. *Transportation of Hazardous Materials.* Washington, DC: U. S. Government Printing Office, OTA Publication No. SET-304, 1986.

Wilson, J. B., S. J. Ventura, L. M. Koonin, and A. M. Spitz. Pregnancy in adolescents. In: *From Data to Action: CDC's Public Health Surveillance for Women, Infants, and Children,* edited by L. S. Wilcox, and J. S. Marks. Atlanta, GA: Centers for Disease Control and Prevention, 1994, pp. 369–379.

4

Monitoring the Health of a Population

OWEN DEVINE
R. GIBSON PARRISH

> Facts which at first seem improbable will even on scant explanation, drop the cloak which has hidden them and stand forth in naked and simple beauty.
>
> —Galileo Galilei (1564–1642)

To react effectively to events affecting the health of a population, public health practitioners must be able to monitor accurately the occurrence and risk factors for disease and injury. This monitoring involves two separate but interdependent efforts: the efficient collection of meaningful measures of the population's risk and the use of suitable methods to evaluate these measures. These two efforts are the focus of this chapter, which covers methodological issues related to both the collection and preliminary evaluation of public health monitoring data. We begin with a discussion of issues related to the efficient collection of information on the health of a target population. We examine the goals of public health monitoring and strategies for identifying and collecting the information necessary to attain those goals. Then we describe a variety of exploratory techniques that are useful in the preliminary analysis of public health monitoring data. The chapter concludes with a brief evaluation of the potential utility of geographic information systems (GIS) as components of public health monitoring systems.

Collection of Public Health Monitoring Data

Monitoring a public health problem requires the collection of information about the affected population, its health problems, and, if known, the causes or risk factors for the health problems. Understanding the relationships between the health problem and its causes is necessary to design the most efficient and effective system for monitoring. A causal pathway for a health problem whose causative agent is environmental is shown in Figure 4.1. If the health problem is well studied and specific intervention or control measures are known, the monitoring should be directed to the point(s) in the pathway closest to the point(s) of control (e.g., monitoring level of air pollutants, monitoring sanitary practices in restaurants, and monitoring immunization coverage). For a newly identified health problem, the causes or risk factors may not be known, and initial monitoring usually will be directed at the health problem itself [e.g., acquired immunodeficiency syndrome (AIDS), eosinophilia-myalgia syndrome (EMS), and Hantavirus]. As a better understanding of the health problem and its causes is developed through etiological studies (see Chapter 5), monitoring can be refined and directed at the most appropriate point(s) in the health problem's causal pathway.

Purpose of Monitoring

Monitoring the health of a population is usually done

- to identify new health problems
- to characterize geographic and demographic distributions of health problems
- to determine temporal trends of known health problems

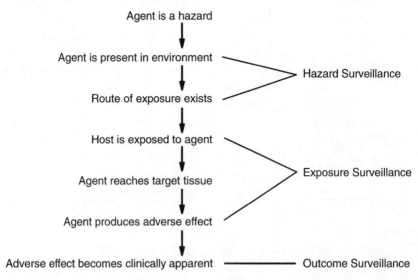

Figure 4.1. The process by which an environmental agent produces an adverse effect and the corresponding types of public health surveillance used for monitoring. [From Thacker et al, 1996.]

- to assess effectiveness of interventions or control measures for a health problem by monitoring the problem or its risk factors or causative agent(s)

Although the basic purposes of monitoring are few, the uses for monitoring data are many and have been well described elsewhere (Institute of Medicine, 1988; Thacker, 1994). The purpose of a particular monitoring system may depend on the level of understanding of a population and its health problems and of the causes of particular health problems. If the population and its health status are well understood, the principal purposes of monitoring would be to assess the effectiveness of interventions or controls and to detect new problems. The approaches for detecting new health problems and assessing effectiveness are different. Detecting new problems usually requires monitoring the *entire* population for significant, new causes of morbidity or mortality. Such monitoring requires the collaboration of primary and specialized health care providers and public health officials at the local, national, and international levels, including the maintenance of a good communication network that allows the timely exchange of information among these parties. In contrast, assessing the effectiveness of interventions can target the affected population rather than the entire population and focus on a specific health problem, its etiological agent, or a modifiable risk factor.

If the population's health status is not well characterized, the initial goal of monitoring would be to identify the health problems and to quantify the geographic and demographic distribution. As the population's health status becomes better defined and etiological studies help identify the causes of the health problems, the purpose of monitoring will shift to monitoring trends of identified health problems over time and the effectiveness of interventions. The purpose of monitoring is *not* etiological research. Nevertheless, monitoring may contribute to the planning and design of etiological studies by (*1*) characterizing certain aspects (e.g., geographic and demographic distribution over time) of a public health problem, (*2*) suggesting hypotheses for etiological studies, and (*3*) identifying populations in which studies should be conducted.

Another critical element of setting up a monitoring system is deciding what will be monitored and developing good working definitions for the objects of the monitoring system (e.g., causal agents, risk factors, and health problems) (Centers for Disease Control and Prevention, 1997). As previously described above, the specificity of the definition may depend on the level of understanding of a health problem and its causes. When a new problem is recognized, the initial working definition may be general and may be a combination of symptoms, signs, or laboratory tests. As the problem and its causes, risk factors, and biological effects are characterized, the definition often becomes more specific. For example, the definition of AIDS used for monitoring has become more specific as the disease has become better understood (Centers for Disease Control and Prevention, 1992).

Information Needed for Monitoring

Once a population, health problem, or risk factor is identified as needing to be monitored, several practical questions must be answered to select the most appropriate method for monitoring, including

- What information is needed on the health problem to assist in public health planning and interventions?
- How quickly is this information needed?
- How long should monitoring continue and what should be the frequency of monitoring (e.g., continuous, periodic)?
- For which population(s) should this information be obtained? Does the entire population need to be monitored or will a sample provide sufficient information?
- What is the quality of the information needed?
- What resources are available for monitoring?
- Who is responsible for monitoring?

Usually, information is needed regarding the geographic extent of the health problem (e.g., county, province, state, country, and world), affected population(s) within this geographic area (e.g., young, elderly, poor, and immunocompromised), and trend over time (e.g., stable, increasing, and erratic). For a new health problem, answers to these questions may be unknown; establishing an intensive, formal monitoring system for the area in which the problem is first identified may be necessary in concert with an additional, less formal effort elsewhere to solicit reports of the problem. As the geographic extent of the problem becomes better characterized, the area covered by the monitoring system should be modified accordingly. For health problems with well-known geographic and demographic distributions, resources should not be expended on areas and populations not affected by the problem. (The monitoring systems set up to identify cases of smallpox during its eradication are a good example of appropriate geographic tailoring of monitoring systems.) Finally, as a health problem is controlled or nears elimination, reducing the resources devoted to its monitoring may be appropriate, so that the resources can be devoted to other, more pressing problems. However, the problem should be adequately monitored to detect quickly any breakdown or failure of the effectiveness of control measures (e.g., tuberculosis in the United States and increased cigarette smoking among teenagers).

For health problems whose incidence changes slowly over time, periodic monitoring of a sample of the affected population may provide sufficient information for public health planning (e.g., heart disease and diet and long-term trends of childhood lead poisoning or birth defects). Conversely, controlling health problems that can spread quickly or unpredictably within a population may require continuous monitoring (Table 4.1) of the entire population (e.g., crack cocaine

Table 4.1. Issues to Consider when Developing a Monitoring System

---

Place:

    Extent of area: county, province, state, country, world

    Entire area, or subsection(s)

Time:

    Frequency: continuous, periodic, one point in time

    Duration: limited, indefinite

Person:

    Population, risk factor, environmental hazard, etiological agent

    Entire population, sample

---

abuse, EMS, meningococcal outbreak, adverse effects from a newly introduced drug, and serious injuries from a newly introduced consumer product such as automobile air bags).

Characteristics of Monitoring Systems

Monitoring systems are distinguished by the following:

- the source of information
- the strategy for obtaining information
- the use of primary or secondary data
- the population coverage

There are two basic *sources of information:* members of the population or their surrogates (e.g., spouse and daughter) and health care providers or their records. For members of the population, information may be obtained through interviewing, soliciting information by using questionnaires or reporting forms, performing physical or laboratory examinations independent of routine health care (e.g., household interview surveys and physical examination surveys), or receiving or abstracting administrative or other nonmedical records.

Information may be obtained from health care providers through interviewing, soliciting information using questionnaires or reporting forms, or reviewing or abstracting their records (e.g., hospital discharge surveys, and birth defects or cancer registries). Some monitoring systems may use a combination of these sources (e.g., vital records systems).

There are two basic *strategies for obtaining information.* First, volunteer or paid agents of the monitoring system can actively and systematically collect data concerning health problems affecting the population (which may be accomplished through the active solicitation of reports of health problems). Second, the population or health care provider can make unsolicited reports concerning the health problem, such as consumer product complaints or reports of adverse effects of drugs or notifiable diseases. Depending on the perceived public health importance of the health problems (e.g., rabies, seasonal upper respiratory infections), and incentives for reporting (e.g., money, professional recognition) or penalties for not reporting the health problem (e.g., fines and professional sanction), the completeness and quality of reporting may vary considerably.

Either of these strategies may involve the collection or use of *primary* or *secondary* data. Primary data consists of new information obtained through observation or interview of, or the completion of forms by, individuals or health care providers. An example of primary data collection is the completion of a death certificate by a funeral director using information obtained from a decedent's family. Secondary data are derived from existing records or information, usually obtained for another purpose. An example of active collection of secondary data is the abstraction of data from medical records for a birth defects registry.

Finally, the extent of *coverage of a population* distinguishes different monitoring systems. A monitoring system may attempt to cover the entire population and all occurrences of the health problem(s) affecting it (e.g., vital records system, cancer registry, census of occupational injuries, and the reporting of notifiable diseases) or only part of the population or some occurrences of the health problem. The latter is usually accomplished through some type of sampling strategy. Samples may be drawn so that they are representative of the population, or they may attempt to obtain information on easily identified occurrences with no effort to ensure completeness or representativeness (e.g., convenience sample and sentinel surveillance). These characteristics and other attributes for six important monitoring systems are shown in Table 4.2.

Whether an existing source of information can be used for monitoring the health problem or a new system must be developed should be determined next. Use of existing information or monitoring system(s) may reduce the cost of monitoring and provide data more quickly but may not provide all the needed information. (See Chapter 3 for a detailed discussion of existing sources of data.) If one existing system does not provide all necessary data, the use of two or more systems may provide sufficient information. Linkage of existing information systems, if feasible, may facilitate this process (Williamson et al., 1995). If health data regarding individuals are needed, legal or ethical considerations concerning individual privacy may either preclude or limit the use or linkage of existing data or the situation may require (*1*) special safeguards for the data, (*2*) legal authority to access data, or (*3*) consent of individuals for the release or use of their health data.

If a new data system is to be developed, all of the previously discussed issues should be considered, given the significant commitment of time, staff, and other resources usually needed. Planning should be undertaken in collaboration with all groups that will be participating in or be affected by the monitoring system to ensure that the system (*1*) is needed, acceptable, and feasible given available resources; and (*2*) will provide the information required to address the public health problem.

Table 4.2. Characteristics of Selected Monitoring Systems

Monitoring System	Source of Information	Strategy	Coverage of Population	Primary or Secondary Data	Cost per Report	Timeliness	Quality of Data	Frequency of Data Collection	Completeness of Coverage
Reports of notifiable diseases	Provider	Passive	Entire	Primary	+	+++	+	++++	+
Breast cancer and birth defects registries	Provider	Active	Entire	Secondary	+++	++	+++	++	+++
Census of Fatal Occupational Injuries (CFOI)	Provider	Active	Entire	Secondary	+++	++	+++	++	+++
Vital records (mortality)	Provider & individual	Passive	Entire	Primary	++	+++	++	++++	++++
National Health Interview Survey (NHIS)	Individual	Active	Sample	Primary	+++	+	+++	++	+++
National Health Examination and Nutrition Survey (NHANES)	Provider & individual	Active	Sample	Primary	++++	+	++++	+	+++

With a clear understanding of the information needed from the monitoring system for public health planning and action, the distinguishing features of different monitoring methods, and the capability of existing sources of information to meet these needs, selecting or designing an appropriate monitoring system should be possible. For example, if high-quality data are required and timeliness and cost are not major considerations, a census or survey is appropriate. For example, the periodic National Health and Nutrition Examination Survey establishes national reference values in the United States for nutritional and physical status. Censuses collect information on all deaths, motor vehicle–related fatalities, and occupation-related fatalities in the United States.

Managing Data

Data for monitoring health problems should be collected, managed, and stored in a systematic way. Although paper forms are still used for several major monitoring systems, the use of computers for collecting, manipulating, and storing electronic data is widespread. The transmission of data should take advantage of existing standards for electronic data interchange (EDI) of health data (e.g., X12, HL7), and data items should be collected, managed, and stored using standard definitions and coding and classification schemes (e.g., SNOMED, ICD), if available and appropriate. Computer software used to collect and manage monitoring data should allow import of data from and export to commonly used database and statistical formats. Proprietary or one-of-a-kind software applications or those with limited import or export capabilities should not be used.

Assessing Quality

Periodic evaluation of monitoring system(s) is important to ensure that needed and useful information is being provided in a timely, cost-effective way (Klaucke, 1994). Assessing the completeness of monitoring data for systems designed to gather all occurrences of a health problem has been done using capture-recapture methods, independent surveys, or linkage methods (Hahn and Stroup, 1994; Dijkhuis et al., 1994).

Exploratory Analysis of Public Health Surveillance Data

Assessing Temporal Trends

The basic approaches to statistical analysis have been presented in Chapter 2. We present here some more advanced techniques of particular value for monitoring.

Typically, public health monitoring data are collected, summarized, and reported over specified time intervals (e.g., weeks, months, or years). The primary goal of exploratory methods applicable to *time series data* is to separate true temporal trends in the underlying risk from the random fluctuations, or "noise," one expects in observable measures of public health. First, the surveyed data should be plotted over the time at which they were collected. For example, Figure 4.2 demonstrates the daily number of emergency room (ER) visits for children aged less than 14 years in four major Atlanta metropolitan hospitals for the summer of 1993. These data indicate an increase in the daily number of ER visits in late spring, midsummer, and early fall. A clearer picture of this possible trend and of meaningful short-term patterns in these data is more evident if the random day-to-day variation in the number of cases is reduced. *Smoothing* potentially highlights meaningful patterns in collections of observed data by reducing the level of random noise.

One of the simplest *smoothers* (mathematical algorithms to attain such noise reduction) is the *moving average*. Suppose surveillance data are collected over time (a *time series*). Summary measures of these data, which we will call Y_i, are associated with a specific time, t_i. As an example, Y_i could be the monthly incidence rate for a specified disease and t_i could designate the month associated with the observed rate. If N such summary measures are included in the series, then Y_i

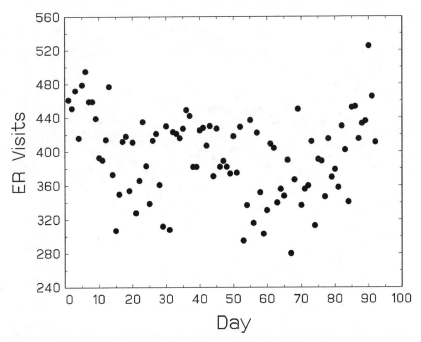

Figure 4.2. Number of pediatric emergency room visits to four metropolitan Atlanta hospitals, June 1–August 31, 1993.

and t_i range from $I = 1$ to $I = N$. To calculate the moving average smoother, the time series is subdivided into N smaller intervals whose length is defined by a user-supplied parameter called the *bandwidth* or, alternatively, the *smoothing window*. If the data are reported daily, (e.g., Fig. 4.2), and the bandwidth is 1 week, the moving average smoother centers each of the N smaller series successively on each t_i so that the smoothing window around each point contains the values observed on the 3 days prior to t_i, the value observed on t_i, and the observations for the 3 days following t_i. Such a collection of values is formed for every day in the series. The moving average smoother value for Y_i is the average of the values falling in the smoothing window centered on t_i, and the smoothed value for Y_i, or $S(Y_i)$, is calculated as:

$$S(Y_i) = \left[\sum_{j=1}^{j=N} I(t_i,t_j) \right]^{-1} \sum_{j=1}^{j=N} t_j \cdot I(t_i,t_j) \qquad [4\text{--}1]$$

where $I(t_i,t_j)$ is an indicator function that takes value one if t_j is included in the smoothing window for t_i and zero if it is not. Figure 4.3 shows the result of applying a moving average smoother on the pediatric ER data with bandwidths of 7 and 21 days. A comparison of the smoothed trend lines illustrates the effect of the bandwidth length on the level of smoothing. The smoother resulting from the 1-

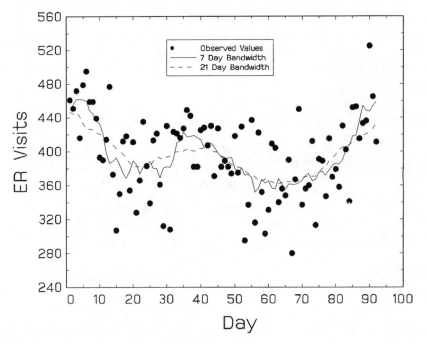

Figure 4.3. Moving average smooths of the pediatric ER data based on 7 and 21 day bandwidths.

week bandwidth retains more of the day-to-day variation in the series than does the smoother based on a 3-week window. The dependence of the amount of smoothing on the bandwidth is an attribute of the moving average smoother and of smoothers in general. Virtually every smoothing approach requires input from the user on the level of smoothing desired. In most cases, this input is a user decision on the number of observations to include in the smoothing window. The smaller the bandwidth, the more local variation is retained. For larger smoothing intervals, local variation is reduced, thus increasing the possibility of highlighting long-term trends. This reduction in random noise, however, may mask potentially meaningful short-term patterns. Approaches for selecting a bandwidth that fits with the analytic goal will be discussed later in this chapter.

Another issue with bandwidth-dependent smoothers concerns the question of how to calculate the smoothed value for time points near the ends of the observed series. The problem with these times is that not enough observations will surround the value to be smoothed to fully complete the smoothing window. For the smoothers presented in Figure 4.3, the available data were used for points near the end of the series. For example, the smoothed value for Y_1, based on a 7 day bandwidth, was computed as the average of Y_1, Y_2, Y_3, and Y_4, whereas the smoothed value at time t_2 was calculated as the average of Y_1, Y_2, Y_3, Y_4, and Y_5. An alternative approach is to reduce the data set so that the first value is no longer Y_1, but rather the first value that will achieve a complete smoothing window. This approach results in exclusion of data near the ends of the observation period which, for large smoothing windows, could be substantial. In addition, whereas this may be an acceptable approach for points near the beginning of the series, the most recently observed values are often of the most interest for monitoring purposes, and discarding these values may not be an attractive alternative. One should remember, however, that if smoothed values near the ends of the series are based on a reduced smoothing window, then these points will have less reduction in random noise than smooth values nearer the center of the series.

The moving average smoother of Equation [4–1] uses equal weights for all observations in the smoothing window. Intuitively, the smoothed value for time t_i should place greater influence on Y_i and values observed close to t_i than on values observed near the ends of the smoothing interval. Differential weighting based on proximity to t_i can be incorporated into the smoother by using a weighted running average where the smoothed value at time t_i is

$$S(Y_i) = \left(\sum_{j=1}^{j=N} w_{ij} \right)^{-1} \sum_{j=1}^{j=N} w_{ij}, Y_j \qquad [4\text{–}2]$$

In the above equation, w_{ij} is the weight associated with each observed value such that w_{ij} is greater than or equal to zero for all observations associated with times within the smoothing window surrounding t_i and w_{ij} is equal to zero for observations outside the window. Usually the value of the weights is based on the amount of time separating t_i and t_j. For example, suppose a difference measure for the time separating t_i and t_j is defined as

$$\Delta_{ij} = \frac{|t_i - t_j|}{C_i + 1}$$

where C_i is the maximum absolute time difference between t_i and the time of any observation falling within the smoothing window. Using Δ_{ij} a weight for the observation taken at time t_j can be defined as

$$\begin{aligned} w_{ij} &= 1 - \Delta_{ij} & \text{if, } \Delta_{ij} < 1 \\ &= 0 & \text{if, } \Delta_{ij} \geq 1 \end{aligned} \qquad\qquad [4\text{--}3]$$

and a weighted average smooth can be calculated using Equation [4–2]. Figure 4.4 compares a weighted running average smooth of the pediatric ER data, based on a 21-day bandwidth with weights given by Equation [4–3], with an unweighted running average smooth derived by using the same length of smoothing window. Although the weighted and unweighted smooths are actually quite similar in this example, there is a tendency for the unweighted smoother to be less resistant (more sensitive) to observations near the ends of the smoothing interval.

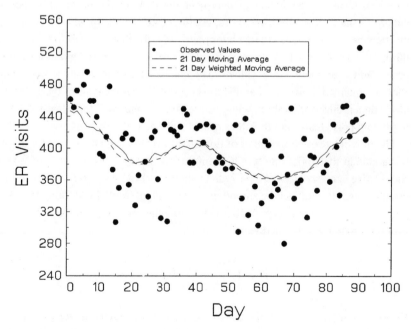

Figure 4.4. Weighted and unweighted moving average smooths of the pediatric ER data based on a 21 day bandwidth.

The weighting function defined in Equation [4–3] is symmetrical about t_i in that the weight assigned to the observation at time t_{i+k} equals the weight given the observation taken at t_{i-k}. Using a symmetrical function to define the weights used in a running weighted average smoother is the basic idea in a collection of approaches known as *kernel smoothers*. The difference between various kernel smoothers is the definition of the formula, called the *kernel function*, used to define the weights. For example, the kernel function in Equation [4–3] is sometimes called a triangle kernel. Another common kernel smoother uses the standard normal probability density function, which is symmetrical, to define the weights such that

$$w_{ij} = \frac{1}{\sqrt{2\pi}\,\sigma}\, e^{\frac{-(ti - t_j)^2}{2\sigma^2}} \qquad [4\text{--}4]$$

where σ is a user-specified constant.

Since the average of a group of numbers can be highly influenced by a few anomalous values, a smoothed value for Y_i more resistant to occasional outliers is obtained using the median of the values with observation times that fall within the smoothing window. For example, Figure 4.5 shows both a *moving median smoother,* based on a 21-day bandwidth, and the corresponding 21-day moving

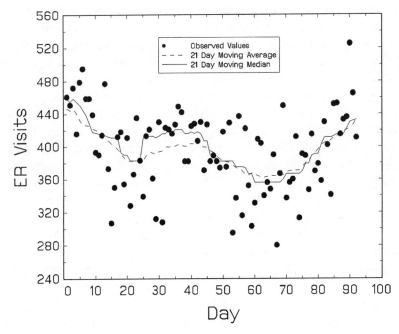

Figure 4.5. Moving median and moving average smooths of the pediatric ER data based on a 21 day bandwidth.

average smooth for the pediatric ER data. Notice the tendency of the median smoother to be less influenced by the occasional unusually low visit counts between days 25 and 45 as compared with the less resistant moving average smooth. As with the average-based smoothers, the moving median smoother requires specification of the bandwidth that will control the level of smoothing applied to the data. Some fixed-bandwidth median-based smoothers, however, are available in which several smooths are applied both to the data and the resulting *residuals*. These residuals are the original observed value minus the current smoothed estimate. The smoothed residuals are then added back to the smoothed estimate in a process known as *twicing* (Tukey, 1977).

As an alternative to using a moving mean or median smoother, a model can be fit to reflect the association between the values in the series and the time of observation. For example, a quadratic equation of the form

$$Y_i = \beta_0 + \beta_1 \cdot t_i + \beta_2 \cdot t_i^2 \qquad [4\text{--}5]$$

(where β_i are coefficients of the model, which will be estimated using the data) could provide an adequate representation of the time trend in the observed data. However, if the series has trends that cannot be modeled by a simple polynomial (e.g., cyclical patterns), then a suitable model for the entire series might be prohibitively complex. Alternatively, the modeling effort could focus on subsets of the series as determined by a selected bandwidth. Within these subintervals, a simple model like the one in Equation [4–5] might adequately describe the short-term trends and provide an acceptable smoothed estimate. One approach to fitting models to successive subsets of the data is called *locally weighted regression smoothing* (Cleveland and Delvin, 1988). To construct such a smoother, a bandwidth surrounding each point in the series is first specified. A model, such as Equation [4–5], is then derived for the collection of times and observed health values that fall within the bandwidth using linear regression techniques. The resulting estimates for the β's are then substituted back into the model to produce a smoothed value for Y_i. As with the moving average smoother, it is reasonable that the smoothed value for Y_i produced by this localized regression should be more heavily influenced by values close to t_i than by values farther away. To incorporate differential weighting, a weighting function can be used to emphasize observations near the middle of the bandwidth in the estimation of the β's. We will assume that the bandwidth is defined to include t_i and its $k - 1$ nearest neighbors so that k observations will be used in the localized fitting procedure. Weights for these k observations are then defined by using a specified symmetrical function (e.g., the normal kernel function of Equation [4–4]). Using these values, a weighted regression can be fit to the collection of data falling within the bandwidth based on, for example, the quadratic model given in Equation [4–5]. The predicted value resulting from this local regression fit can then be used as a

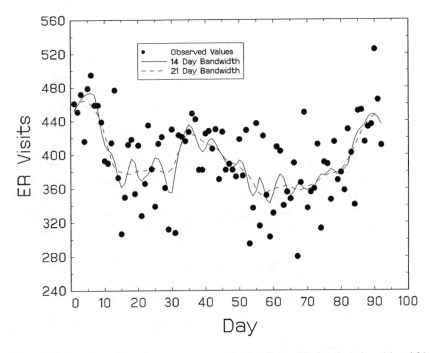

Figure 4.6. Locally weighted regression smooth of pediatric ER data based on 14 and 21 day bandwidths.

smoothed value for Y_i. Figure 4.6 shows the result of using a local regression smoother on the pediatric ER data with bandwidths equal to 14 and 21 days. The weights in this smooth correspond to the normal kernel function of Equation [4–4].

These cursory descriptions of a collection of approaches useful to smooth time-series data do not determine which method is best for exploratory analysis of public health monitoring data. In most cases, weighted moving average, moving median, and locally weighted regression approaches are likely to produce similar smooths if based on comparable bandwidths. Selection of the bandwidth is the primary consideration when using these types of smoothers, although some methods for automatic bandwidth selection are available (MathSoft, 1995). Given the relative simplicity of producing the types of smooths, however, bandwidth selection can be approached iteratively. For example, a user can try a variety of bandwidths and then make a decision as to which level of smoothing best addresses the trade-off between oversmoothing and variance reduction in light of the particular monitoring question.

The methods for initial evaluations of time trends can be followed by additional modeling efforts based on *time-series analysis techniques.* For example, an *autoregressive model* that has the form

$$Y_i = \beta_1 \cdot Y_{i-1} + \beta_2 \cdot Y_{i-2} + \beta_k \cdot Y_{i-k} + \epsilon_i \qquad\qquad [4\text{--}6]$$

could be fit to the data where Y_i is the observed value at time t_i, Y_{i-k} is the value observed at time t_{i-k}; ϵ_i is an error term; and $\beta_1, \beta_2, \ldots, \beta_k$ are unknown parameters. Alternatively, the model in Equation [4–6] could be augmented into what is called an *autoregressive moving average* (ARIMA) model by adding a linear combination of random error terms associated with each time used in the estimation of Y_i (Box and Jenkins, 1976). Several methods are available for estimating the parameters of these models based on the observed series of data (Fuller, 1996). In these approaches, however, estimation of the model parameters must account for the serial correlation likely to be present in the data. A useful advantage of this modeling approach is the ability to forecast future values for the indicator of interest and, also, estimates of uncertainty of these forecasts. Alternative approaches to time-series analysis are available to modeling serially correlated health indicator data. For example, generalized regression methods (Zeger, 1988; Singh and Roberts, 1992) and Bayesian state space modeling (Berzuini and Larizza, 1996) have been applied to analysis of serially collected health data.

Assessing Spatial Trends

Using maps to illustrate the geographic distribution of disease has a long history in epidemiological research (Gilbert, 1958). The most common types of maps used for these purposes are *chloropleth* (or *thematic*) *maps* and *dot density maps.* Thematic maps provide geographic summaries of measures of disease burden associated with specified areas (e.g., zip codes, counties, or states). For example, absolute area-specific measures such as disease counts; prevalence, incidence, or mortality rates; or relative measures [e.g., relative risks and standardized mortality ratios (SMR)] often are illustrated using thematic maps (Devine at al., 1991). Sometimes the summary measure shown on a thematic map is related to the probability of observing a measure at least the size of that seen in each area under a set of distributional assumptions (Pickle et al., 1987). As an example of thematic mapping, Figure 4.7 shows a county-based map of age-adjusted lung cancer mortality rates for Ohio for the years 1968–1994. Usually, user-specified categories of the mapped values are determined to subdivide the areas into, potentially, meaningful groups. In Figure 4.7, the age-adjusted rates have been stratified into three categories: those counties with rates in the lowest 25% of the state, those with rates from 26% through 75%, and those areas with observed incidence rates in the highest 25% in the state. This categorization focuses on an internal comparison of Ohio counties. Alternatively, one categorization could be based on external reference values such as rates across all United States counties. The num-

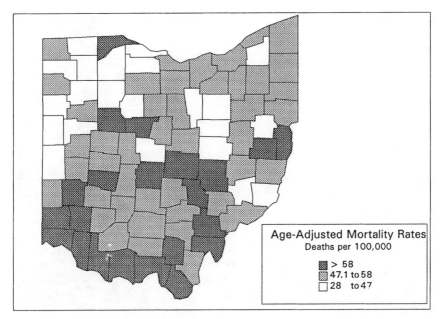

Figure 4.7. Age-adjusted lung cancer mortality rates for counties in the state of Ohio, 1968–1994.

ber and definition of categories used in a thematic map are parameters that re-quire careful thought and should be based on a clear a priori specification of the geographic information the mapper wishes to extract.

The second type of map commonly employed in public health applications is the dot density map. Figure 4.8 contains a dot density map in which the stars rep-resent the address at time of death for a collection of persons who died between 1958 and 1992 and had lung cancer listed as the primary cause of death. In gen-eral, dot density maps are based on a one-to-one matching between the number of events and the number of points. However, most mapping software allows for many-to-one matching (i.e., one point can represent a number of health events). Examination of this map might lead one to suspect increased lung cancer risk in the eastern portion of the region being considered, which corresponds to the west-ern edges of the city of Cincinnati, Ohio. The apparent increase in risk in the map in Figure 4.8, however, is more likely a reflection of higher population density closer to the metropolitan Cincinnati area. Although the need to adjust for nonuniform population distribution seems obvious, this characteristic of disease-event mapping often leads to misinterpretation of dot density maps even by trained epidemiologists. As a result, most public health mapping applications use thematic mapping of area-based summary measures (e.g., incidence rates) that can be adjusted to remove the effects of differing population size.

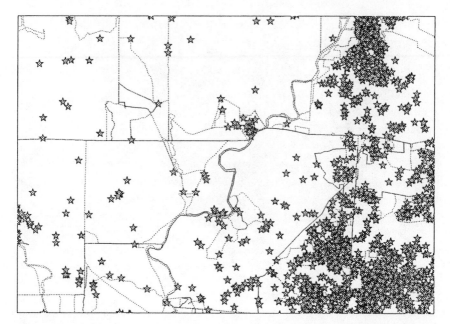

Figure 4.8. Addresses at time of death for individuals with lung cancer listed as the primary cause of death in portions of Hamilton and Butler Counties, Ohio, 1958–1992.

A troublesome limitation of thematic mapping for public health is the reliance on political as opposed to etiological definition of areas. Another type of mapping that may address this problem is called *contour mapping* (Carrat and Valleron, 1992). Contour maps are produced by interpolating values for the monitoring indicator of interest between areas where the measures have been collected and then drawing a series of lines, called *isopleths,* connecting locations with similar interpolated values. The interpolation methods used to produce contour maps rely on spatial prediction methods (Cressie, 1991). Because the interpolation method used can influence the resulting map and because some mapping software allows creation of contour maps using default prediction methods (Golden Software, 1994), a priori consideration should be given when producing contour maps as to the method of interpolation to be used.

Just as with time-series data, smoothing approaches can reduce the random noise in maps of observable measures of public health. In thematic mapping, where a trade-off exists between geographic resolution and the variability of the mapped estimates, the variance associated with a measure observed in an area tends to increase as the population size in the area decreases (Devine et al., 1994). As a result, highlighted areas on the map may appear to have high risk purely as a result of a small number of inhabitants. This issue can be addressed by combining areas into larger regions. This solution, however, comes at the cost of geographic resolution perhaps to the point where the map is no longer informative. Alternatively, one could apply smoothing approaches to spatially aligned data to reduce random noise and highlight meaningful geographic patterns in the underlying risk. We will discuss two general types of spatial smoothers, nonparametric smoothers and parametric smoothers or, specifically, Bayes and empirical Bayes smooths.

We will first address *nonparametric approaches* to smoothing spatially aligned data in which no particular assumptions are made on the distribution of the observed data. An obvious first choice for a spatial smoother is a weighted average approach. For spatial smoothing, however, a circular, or disk, smoothing window is used as opposed to the linear interval used in smoothing time series. Once this window is defined, the smoothed value is calculated for the region in the center of the disk by using the observed values in areas within a specified distance. As an alternative to defining the smoothing window based on distance, we could calculate the smoothed value for area i, as the weighted average of those areas that share a common boundary with the target area. Regardless of the method for inclusion in the smoothing disk, the smoothed value for area i, where $i = 1, 2, \ldots N$, is defined as

$$S(Y_i) = \left[\sum_{j=1}^{j=N} w_{ij}\, I(i,j) \right]^{-1} \sum_{j=1}^{j=N} w_{ij}\, Y_j\, I(i,j) \qquad [4\text{--}7]$$

where $I(i,j)$ is an indicator function that takes value one if area j is included in the smoothing disk surrounding area i and zero otherwise. The weights used in Equation [4–7] usually are functions of the distance separating the centroids of areas i and j, which we will call d_{ij}, such as $w_{ij} = 1/d_{ij}$ or $w_{ij} = 1/d_{ij}^2$.

As with the one-dimensional time-series smoothers, care must be taken when smoothing observations associated with areas near the map boundaries. One approach to addressing the boundary problem is to include information from surrounding areas outside the region of interest to complete the smoothing window for border regions. In some cases (e.g., if the boundary is an ocean), this approach may not be feasible. Alternatively, one could just fill the smoothing window with as much information as is available. In this case, because smoothed values for border areas are based on the average of a smaller number of neighbors, the stabilizing effects of the smoothing process will be reduced along the map edges.

As with the temporal smoothers, the sensitivity of the spatial smoothing procedure to outliers may be reduced by basing the smoother on medians as opposed to means. In Figure 4.9, two smoothed maps of Ohio lung cancer data illustrate median-based disk smoothing. Figure 4.9A was developed using a smoothing disk that incorporates all areas with centroids within 100 miles of the area being smoothed. Figure 4.9B is a similar median smoothed map but with smoothing neighborhoods based on a disk radius of 50 miles. The difference in the level of smoothing between the two maps, again, illustrates the effect of the number of neighbors used in calculating the smoothed value on the amount of local variation retained.

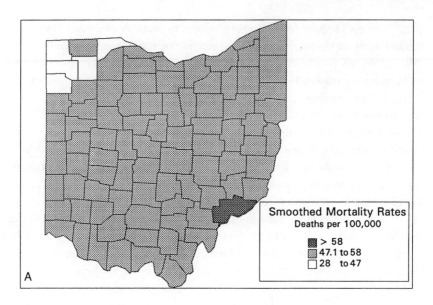

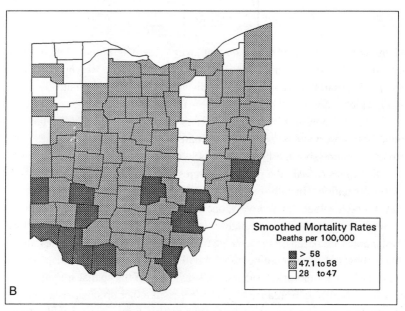

Figure 4.9. Median-based smooths of age-adjusted lung cancer mortality rates for counties in the state of Ohio, 1968–1994, using smoothing windows for (*A*) 100 and (*B*) 50 miles.

As an alternative to the distance and adjacency criteria, the smoothing window could be defined to include a specified number of neighbors of area i. For example, one could base the smoothed value for each area on the median of the observed value in that area and the values observed in the k closest areas to the one being smoothed. Consider the following example of such a k *nearest-neighbor* *approach.* To obtain a smoothed value for area i, the $N - 1$ candidate areas to be included in the window, N total areas minus the area we are smoothing, should be ranked by their distance from area i. Let Y_1^* be the observed value in the area located the minimum distance from area i, Y_2^* be the value associated with the area having the second smallest distance from area i, and Y_{N-1}^* be the value observed in the area located the farthest from the target area. Using a k nearest-neighbor median smoother, the smoothed value for area i is defined as

$$S(Y_i) = \text{Median}\ (Y_i, Y_1^*, Y_2^*, Y_3^*, \dots, Y_k^*) \qquad [4\text{--}8]$$

This nearest-neighbor definition of the smoothing neighborhood is useful when the areas to be mapped differ significantly in geographic size. For example, in smoothing county level measures across the entire United States, a distance-based definition of the smoothing window can lead to a map in which the number of observations used to calculate the smoothed values can differ substantially across areas.

In both the observed (Fig. 4.7) and 50 mile median smoothed (Fig. 4.9B) maps of the Ohio lung cancer data, there may be a suggestion of a gradient in the rates from north-northeast towards the south. In this situation, a distance-only definition of the smoothing neighborhood may not be the best criterion for designating the smoothing window. An alternative median-based smoothing procedure called *headbanging* (Tukey and Tukey, 1981) allows directional as well as proximity constraints to be placed on the definition of the smoothing window. Empirical evidence indicates that the method provides a good balance between smoothing random noise and maintaining certain types of spatial patterns (Hansen, 1991). Another smoothing approach, called *median polish,* reduces local random variation while maintaining linear spatial trends by modeling observed values based on the relative locations of the areas in which they were observed (Cressie, 1991). To implement the median polish smoother, a grid system is imposed on the map such that each area is assigned to a specific intersection of vertical and horizontal lines on the grid. Then the observed value in area i, Y_i, is renamed as Y_{lk}, where l and k are the grid coordinates of the intersection closest to the center of area i. If the regions are irregularly spaced or vary substantially in size, assignment of areas to specific grid intersections may be difficult. Once the areas are indexed by grid location, a smoothed value for Y_{lk} is obtained using the model

$$S(Y_{lk}) = m + \alpha_l + \gamma_k \qquad [4\text{--}9]$$

where m is the overall median, α_l is the lth row effect and γ_k is the kth column effect. Estimates of the parameters in Equation [4–9] are obtained by repeated subtraction of row and column medians from each value until convergence. Once the parameter estimates are obtained, the smoothed value, $S(Y_{lk})$, can be substituted for Y_{lk} on the map and median polish residuals can be calculated as

$$r_{lk} = Y_{lk} - S(Y_{lk}) \qquad\qquad [4\text{--}10]$$

These residuals can be useful for analyses that require an adjustment to the observed values that removes large-scale spatial trends (Cressie and Read, 1989).

So far, we have presented spatial smoothing methods that utilize only the empirical evidence presented by the collection of observed area-specific measures. However, in some monitoring applications, the mapper may have some a priori assumption on what the true distribution of disease risk across areas should be. This prior information can then be combined with observed data leading to a *Bayesian* approach to mapping observed measures of public health (Devine et al., 1995). The underlying assumption of the Bayesian approach is that the number of disease events occurring in area i is a realization of a two-stage process. First, each area is subject to an unobservable risk, which for area i we will designate as θ_i. The distribution of these underlying risks across areas, called the *prior distribution,* is the true, but unfortunately unobservable, geographic variation in risk. The observed number of health events, Y_i, is a realization of a second sampling stage that depends on area i's underlying risk. To illustrate, if the distribution of true risks for a given disease across all counties in the United States follows a normal distribution with mean μ and variance γ^2, a histogram of these values would approximate a normal distribution with the given mean and variance. If one area, area i, has true risk θ_i sampled from this normal prior, the number of disease events observed in area i could be assumed to be a Poisson random variable with mean $N_i \cdot \theta_i$ where N_i is the person time at risk observed in area i. In many cases, the Bayes estimate for θ_i has the form

$$\beta(\theta_i) = f(N_i, \gamma^2) \cdot \frac{Y_i}{N_i} + [1 - f(N_i, \gamma^2)] \cdot \mu \qquad\qquad [4\text{--}11]$$

In this estimator, $f(N_i, \gamma^2)$ is a function of N_i and γ^2 that gets close to zero when N_i is small and close to one when N_i is large. Therefore, when N_i is small, and the observed rate, Y_i/N_i, is expected to be unstable, the Bayes estimator gets close to the assumed prior mean, μ. Alternatively, if the observed rate is based on a large value for N_i, indicating that Y_i/N_i is likely to be stable, then the Bayes estimator approaches the observed rate. In general, a Bayes estimator is a weighted average of the observed data and our prior expectations with weights depending on the variability expected in these two values.

The Bayesian approach to mapping public health measurements requires the user to specifiy information (e.g., the values of μ and γ^2 in Equation [4–11]) to summarize his or her prior beliefs about the distribution of risk. The manner in which this information is derived distinguishes the Bayes from the *empirical Bayes* approach (Bernardinelli and Montomoli, 1992). Under a Bayesian approach, the parameters could either be assumed to be known or they can be derived by considering the parameters themselves to be random variables drawn from higher stage sampling distributions called hyperpriors (Mollie, 1996). In the empirical Bayes approach, the values for the unknown parameters are estimated based on the observed data (Clayton and Kaldor, 1987). To illustrate empirical Bayes smoothing, we return to the Ohio county-level lung cancer mortality rates. Suppose we make the assumption that the collection of unobservable risks reflected in the observed rates of Figure 4.7 follow a γ distribution (Evans et al., 1993). In addition, we will assume that the observed number of lung cancer deaths in each county is a Poisson random variable with mean and variance equal to $N_i \cdot \alpha\beta$, where α and β are the unknown parameters of our assumed γ prior distribution on the risk. In this case, the empirical Bayes estimator for the risk in area i is given by

$$EB(\theta_i) = W_i^* \cdot \frac{Y_i}{N_i} + (1 - W_i^*) \cdot \alpha^* \beta^* \qquad [4\text{--}12]$$

where

$$W_i^* = \frac{\beta^* N_i}{\beta^* N_i + 1}$$

and α^* and β^* are estimates of the prior parameters developed from the data. Note that W_i^* is a function of these estimates and that county population size balances the empirical Bayes estimate between the observed rate and the prior expectation depending on the magnitude of N_i.

The choice between a fully bayesian and an empirical Bayes approach involves the user's feelings on using the data to estimate unknown information. While the computational difficulties inherent in a fully Bayesian approach are substantial, a major advantage of this method is that it provides acceptable estimators for the standard error of the smoothed rates. While obtaining the estimates themselves is usually easier under an empirical Bayes approach, getting reasonable estimates of the standard errors associated with the empirical Bayes estimates can be difficult (Louis, 1991). Readers interested in using an empirical Bayes approach that includes estimation of the standard errors should consult a number of references including Kass and Steffey (1989), and Carlin and Gelfand (1990).

Another potential difficulty with both the Bayes and empirical Bayes estimators is that the collection of estimates can actually be too smooth. This oversmoothing is illustrated by the fact that the histogram of a collection of Bayes or empirical Bayes estimates is likely to be narrower than the histogram of the true underlying risks. Oversmoothing can be addressed using what are called *constrained Bayes methods* (Ghosh, 1992; Louis, 1984; Devine and Louis, 1994). These constrained approaches provide almost the stabilization of regular Bayes and empirical Bayes methods but produce collections of estimates with histograms that better approximate the assumed prior distribution.

So far in our consideration of Bayesian smoothing methods, we have made the simplifying, and likely unrealistic, assumption that the collection of area-specific summary measures are independent. In other words, we have assumed that there is no association between the incidence rate observed in area i and the incidence rates occurring in the surrounding areas. This assumption may be unrealistic in that areas close to each other are likely to have similar health data and that this association is likely to decrease with distance. Distance-dependent correlation among both the underlying risks and the observed values can be incorporated into a Bayesian smoothing approach. One way to incorporate this dependence is to develop estimates that are weighted averages of the observed values and a local as opposed to global prior expectation (Marshall, 1991a). As an alternative, one could incorporate a correlation structure into the assumptions on the distributions of both the underlying risk and observed measures (Mollie and Richardson, 1991). The key in deriving Bayes and empirical Bayes estimators when one assumes spatial dependence is to postulate a model for the correlation structure in terms of a relatively small number of parameters (Devine et al., 1994).

Bayesian methods for smoothing maps can be extended to evaluate potential spatial associations between possible predictors of risk and the area-specific realizations of disease impact. For example, if the underlying risk for area i depends on some observable value, X_i then $\alpha\beta$ in Equation [4–12] can be replaced by the model:

$$\mu_i = \lambda_0 + \lambda_1 X_i + \epsilon_i \qquad [4\text{–}13]$$

where γ_0 and γ_1 are unknown parameters and ϵ_i is a random variable term with expected value zero and a specified variance. In addition, a spatial correlation structure can be modeled by assuming that the covariance between ϵ_i and ϵ_j, where ϵ_j is the error term associated with another area, has a specified structure. As when we assumed the prior mean to be constant, the unknown parameters needed to drive the estimates can be obtained under either a fully Bayes or empirical Bayes approach. The type of approach, sometimes called *spatiotemporal modeling* (Waller et al., 1997), allows model-based evaluations of possible associations between disease risk and suspected causative factors.

Assessing Spatiotemporal Dependence in Public Health Monitoring Data

In the previous section, we discussed the likely existence of correlation in collections of spatially or temporally aligned public health surveillance data. In fact, most of the smoothing approaches discussed here are based on an underlying assumption of this dependence as illustrated by their use of localized smoothing windows. The level and structure of this correlation can also have major implica-

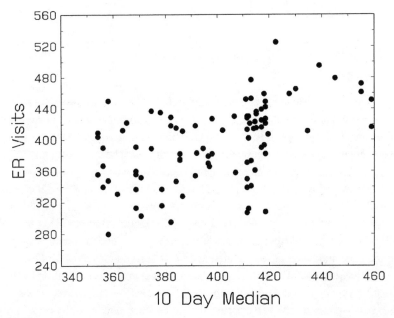

Figure 4.10. Number of pediatric ER visits over the median number of visits in the 10 preceding days and the 10 following days.

tions on the complexity of analyses based on these types of data. As a result, preliminary evaluation of the amount of dependence evident in public health surveillance data can be an important first step in meaningful analysis. The first, but often neglected, step in such an evaluation is to plot the data. For example, *time-lagged plots* can be quite useful in assessing the level of temporal dependence. Figure 4.10 contains a time lag plot for the pediatric ER visit data that illustrates the association between the number of visits on a given day and the median number of visits on the 10 days preceding and following that day. This type of plot can be quite useful for guiding analysis decisions (e.g., selection of a meaningful bandwidth). The spatial equivalent of this type of plot is sometimes referred to as a *nearest neighbor plot* (Haining, 1990), which facilitates examination of the association between the observed value in an area and the median of the values observed in that area's k nearest neighbors.

An extension of this graphic approach, which originated in geostatistics, is called the *variogram* (Cressie, 1991). To produce a variogram, one first creates categories based on the distances separating the areas under consideration. For example, one might create k distinct distance categories depending on d_{ij} such that, if d_{ij} is reasonably close to a value h, the distance separating these areas is placed into category h. If the total number of areas is N, the variogram for areas falling in distance category h given by

$$2\,\gamma(h) = \frac{1}{\displaystyle\sum_{i=1}^{N}\sum_{j=1}^{i} I(d_{ij} = h)} \sum_{i=1}^{N}\sum_{j=1}^{i} (Y_i - Y_j)^2\, I(d_{ij} = h) \qquad [4\text{--}14]$$

where $2\gamma(h)$ is the value of the variogram at distance h and $I(d_{ij} = h)$ is an indicator function that takes value one if d_{ij} falls in category h and zero otherwise. This definition of the variogram is approximately the average squared difference in the observed values among areas separated by distance h. The value of the variogram should be lower for small values of h and should increase with distance up to the point that the observed values are virtually independent. As a result, variograms are useful in determining meaningful radii for smoothing disks and in addressing the adequacy of proposed models for the correlation structure (Devine et al., 1991). The theoretical interpretation of the variogram depends on an assumption that the expected value of the difference of the observed measures for any two areas and the variance of that difference does not depend on the location of the areas under consideration. If this assumption is violated—for example, if there is a large-scale spatial trend in risk across the areas—then one should model the spatial trend in the data, perhaps using a median polish, and then estimate the variogram using the residuals from this fit as the observed data (Cressie and Read, 1989).

As an alternative to graphical summaries of the level of correlation present in surveillance data, test statistics could be used to assess potential dependence. For example, the *autocovariance* and *autocorrelation functions* can be estimated from serially collected observed values to provide an indication of the level of temporal dependence in time-series data (Fuller, 1996). In addition, the *Durbin Watson* and *Moran's I* statistics (Haining, 1990) are used to estimate the potential correlation in temporally and spatially aligned observations. Whereas a statistic-based approach provides a summary measure of the level of correlation present in a collection of data, these statistics provide limited insight into the structure of the potential dependency as compared to the graphical methods.

Detection of Aberrations in Public Health Surveillance Data

The detection of aberrations, or clusters, is often a primary consideration when evaluating public health monitoring data. A debate exists, however, about the utility or even the advisability of applying cluster detection methods (Rothman, 1990). We will attempt to avoid this debate by framing our discussion of cluster detection methods purely in the light of exploratory analyses which may, or may not, lead to further more in-depth investigations. Given the increasing geographic specificity of many surveillance systems, however, and availability of software employing spatial analysis methods (Biomedware, 1994), it is likely that the use of cluster detection methods will become a more common component in public health surveillance systems.

The term "unusual clustering" of disease events in space and/or time is not well defined. Besag and Newell (1991) have presented a useful categorization of clustering models into two groups—general and focused clustering. General cluster detection methods are geared towards detection of aggregations of disease events that are unusually close to each other in space, time, or both dimensions. Alternatively, focused clustering methods are directed towards detection of unusual aggregations of disease events relative to a specified location. Cluster detection methods can be further subdivided into those that evaluate the temporal/spatial distribution of aggregate area measures (e.g., incidence rates) and those for evaluation of disease event data based on the specific locations of individuals with the disease of interest.

Reviews of both generalized and focused cluster detection methods are available [e.g., Marshall (1991b), and Waller and Jacquez (1995)]. A few general points concerning cluster detection methods, however, are worth mention. First, if one looks for a cluster long enough, using enough data and many tests, one will find it. This multiple comparison problem is familiar to most epidemiologists. Many cluster detection algorithms involve evaluation of the probability of the observed disease measure under a null hypothesis of constant underlying risk across space and time. Repeated application of these tests to surveillance data, especially across a substantial number of areas, will invariably lead to spurious identification of "clusters" even when the risk is truly constant. Another problem with cluster evaluations is the interpretation of results in that the analyses are likely based on aggregate measures of disease burden (e.g., county incidence rates). This dependence on aggregated data requires that cluster detection methods be considered as ecological analyses with all the inherent drawbacks of this type of approach (Greenland, 1992). As a result, these analyses must be interpreted as purely exploratory, and the appropriate presentation is likely to be of equal or greater complexity than derivation of the result itself. The availability of more precise geographic location data on location of cases (e.g., address at time of diagnosis) in combination with the use of GIS, however, can lead to more powerful evaluations of potential spatial trends [e.g., using the case-control approach of Cuzick and Edwards (1990)].

Given these caveats, we will, for the sake of illustration, evaluate an a priori spatial hypothesis on the distribution of lung cancer risk in Ohio. Figure 4.11 shows the observed age-adjusted lung cancer mortality rates examined earlier along with the location of the Fernald Feed Material Processing Center (FMPC). The FMPC, a component of the United States nuclear weapons production complex, operated as a uranium processing facility from 1952 through 1989. Al-

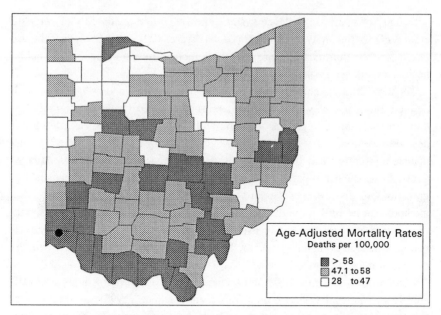

Figure 4.11. Age-adjusted lung cancer mortality rates for counties in the state of Ohio, 1968–1994. Circle marks location of the former feed materials production center.

though there was never a nuclear reactor at the facility, uranium ore was processed into target elements on the site. In the course of this production, uranium dust, radon, and radon-decay products were released into the atmosphere and may have contaminated the community surrounding the site (Radiological Assessments Corporation, 1996). Therefore, the distribution of lung cancer risk is important, since lung cancer is the most likely outcome of exposure to these contaminants. We will employ a focused clustering procedure (Stone, 1988) to evaluate lung cancer mortality relative to the site. Stone's procedure is based on the assumption that, if the counties surrounding the FMPC were arranged in increasing distance from the site, where area l is the closest and area k is the farthest away, then the expected number of lung cancer deaths in any area, say $E[Y_i]$, can be modeled as

$$E[Y_i] = \lambda_i \, \gamma \, N_i \qquad\qquad [4\text{--}15]$$

where N_i is the person time at risk in area i, γ is the average true risk across all areas, and γ_i is the change in the average risk due to being in area i. Estimators for the γ_i's are derived using *isotonic regression,* which is a *maximum likelihood* approach under the constraint that the estimated value for γ_i must be as large or larger than the estimated value for γ_j if area i is closer to the FMPC than is area j. The probability of observing the collection of estimated γ_i's derived from the ob-

served rates can be estimated by using a *Monte Carlo process*, in which the observed total number of lung cancer deaths are repeatedly distributed across counties under the null spatial hypothesis that γ_i equals one for all i. This simulation-
based variation of Stone's test is used because of the relatively low power of the
original approach (Bithell, 1992). In Figure 4.12, those areas with estimated relative risks higher than the 95th percentile of the distribution of expected estimates
under the null hypothesis are highlighted. Multiple comparison problems are reduced in this modified approach by only drawing the map illustrating the simula-
tion based county-level p-values when an overall likelihood ratio test is significant at the 0.05 level. The results of this evaluation indicate a grouping of
estimated increased risk areas in the vicinity of the Fernald plant. However, this
analysis takes no account of smoking prevalance, the primary risk factor for lung
cancer, and to the fact that the areas with estimated elevated risk tend to be close
to the Kentucky border, a state with one of the highest estimated smoking preva-
lences in the United States (Shopland et al., 1996). Perhaps further investigation
of the distribution of lung cancer risk relative to the FMPC site is warranted
(Waller et al., 1997), but these analyses are by no means conclusive.

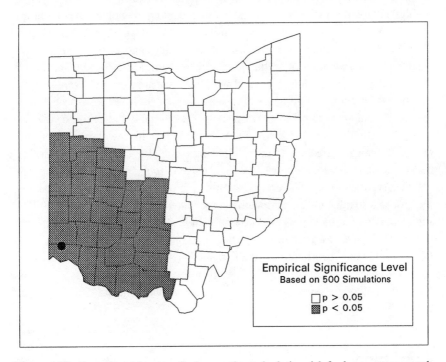

Figure 4.12. Counties with unusually large estimated relative risk for lung cancer mortality based on a modified Stone's test, Ohio, 1968–1994. Circle marks location of the former
feed materials production center.

Applications of Geographic Information Systems

Mapping has been an important part of analysis of public health data for hundreds of years. The advent of GIS, however, has the potential to extend geographic analysis of health data beyond the production of static maps. Although many public health professionals are aware of the existence and the basic principles underlying GIS programs, the utility of this technology in terms of application to monitoring systems is still in the developmental stage (Waller and McMaster, 1996).

Geographic information systems are computer programs that allow users to display and manipulate spatially referenced data. Mapping is one of the most important utilities of GIS in public health surveillance. The ability to produce maps quickly is a first step in exploratory spatial analysis. The true strength of GIS, however, comes through allowing interaction between the mapper and the spatially referenced data due to the storage of data in *layers*. Layers are collections of georeferenced information separated and stored in different groups. For example, in the lung cancer incidence map of Figure 4.8, the geographic boundaries of the municipalities are one layer, while the actual location of lung cancer deaths is stored in another. The ability to overlay different layers on the same map can highlight potential spatial associations possibly leading to etiological hypotheses. In addition, because of the link between the recorded data and geographic locations, information can be retrieved from the data tables underlying the map using spatial queries. Examples of spatial queries include pointing to a particular case in Figure 4.8 and having data associated with that case appear on the screen or requesting information on all cases that occur within 5 miles of a suspected point source of contamination. Most GIS packages also enable buffering, or the creation of new regions around specified locations. This buffering capability can create regions not associated with the original data scale. Layering, spatial querying, and spatial data manipulation can provide powerful tools for evaluation of public health surveillance data. The drawback, however, of most commercially available GIS packages is that these manipulative procedures are the limit of their capabilities. In particular, most packages do not include algorithms for exploratory spatial analysis. One way to address this shortcoming is to develop an interfacing capability allowing incorporation of these methods within a GIS. Alternatively, some GIS packages are developing links to software that will increase the capability for spatial analysis relevant to evaluations of public health (Kaluzny et al., 1996).

Conclusion

Throughout this chapter, several issues have been addressed that concern both the collection and exploratory analysis of monitored public health surveillance data.

These preliminary investigations are important for several reasons including early detection of possible aberrations, evaluation of temporal or spatial trends, and, potentially, generation of etiological hypotheses for further investigation. The cursory nature of the methods presented, although useful for exploratory analysis, must be kept in mind throughout the monitoring process. Observation of an unusual aggregation of disease events in the vicinity of a nuclear facility, although of interest to the public health professional, certainly is not proof of causation or even association. However, such an aggregation is likely to come to the attention of the media and concerned citizens, and quick response to this concern depends on effective methods for evaluating monitored data.

Thus, this chapter aims to either illustrate or provide references to methods that can be implemented in federal, state, and local public health agencies at nominal cost in terms of software and statistical complexity. As the spatial and temporal resolution of available public health surveillance data increases, these methods will provide tools allowing public health professionals to effectively utilize these data to better monitor the health of their constituents.

References

Bernardinelli, L., and C. Montomoli. Empirical Bayes versus fully bayesian analysis of geographic variation in disease risk. *Stat. Med.* 11:983–1007, 1992.

Berzuini, C., and C. Larizza. A unified approach for modeling longitudinal and failure time data, with application in medical monitoring. *IEEE Trans. Pattern Anal. Mach. Intellig.* 18:109–123, 1996.

Besag, J., and J. Newell. The detection of clusters in rare diseases. *J. R. Stat. Soc.* 154:143–155, 1991.

Biomedware. *Stat! Statistical Software for the Clustering of Health Events.* Ann Arbor, MI: Biomedware, 1994.

Bithell, J. Statistical methods for analyzing point-source exposures. In: *Geographical and Environmental Epidemiology: Methods for Small-Area Studies,* edited by P. Elliot, J. Cuzick, D. English, and R. Stern. New York: Oxford University Press, 1992.

Box, G., and G. Jenkins. *Time Series Analysis: Forecasting and Control.* Oakland, CA: Holden-Day, 1976.

Carlin, B., and A. Gelfand. Approaches for empirical Bayes confidence intervals. *J. Am. Stat. Assoc.* 84:105–114, 1990.

Carrat, F., and A. Valleron. Epidemiologic mapping using the "kriging" method: application to an influenza-like illness epidemic in France. *Am. J. Epidemiol.* 135:1293–1300, 1992.

Centers for Disease Control and Prevention. 1993 Revised classification system for HIV infection and expanded surveillance case definition for AIDS among adolescents and adults. *MMWR Morb. Mortal. Wkly. Rep.* 41(RR-17):1–19, 1992.

Centers for Disease Control and Prevention. 1997 Case definitions for infectious conditions under public health surveillance. *MMWR Morb. Mortal. Wkly. Rep.* 46(RR-10):1–55, 1997.

Clayton, D., and J. Kaldor. Empirical Bayes estimates of age-standardized relative risks. *Biometrics* 43:671–681, 1987.

Cleveland, W., and S. Devlin. Locally weighted regression: an approach to regression by local fitting. *J. Am. Stat. Assoc.* 83:596–610, 1988.

Cressie, N. *Statistics for Spatial Data.* New York: John Wiley & Sons, 1991.

Cressie, N., and T. Read. Spatial data analysis of regional counts. *Biometric. J.* 6:699–719, 1989.

Cuzick, J., and R. Edwards. Spatial clustering for inhomogeneous populations. *J. R. Stat. Soc.* 52:73–104, 1990.

Devine, O., J. Annest, M. Kirk, P. Holmgreen, and S. Emrich. *Injury Mortality Atlas of the United States, 1979–1987.* Atlanta, GA: Centers for Disease Control, 1991.

Devine, O. J., and T. A. Louis. A constrained empirical Bayes estimator for incidence rates in areas with small populations. *Stat. Med.* 13:1119–1133, 1994.

Devine, O. J., T. A. Louis, and M. E. Halloran. Empirical Bayes estimators for spatially correlated incidence rates. *Environmetrics* 5:381–398, 1994.

Devine, O. J., T. A. Louis, and M. E. Halloran. Empirical Bayes methods for stabilizing incidence rates before mapping. *Epidemiology* 5:622–630, 1995.

Dijkhuis, H., C. Zwerling, G. Parrish, T. Bennett, and H. C. Kemper. Medical examiner data in injury surveillance: a comparison with death certificates. *Am. J. Epidemiol.* 139(6):637–643, 1994.

Evans, M., N. Hastings, and B. Peacock. *Statistical Distributions.* New York: John Wiley & Sons, 1993.

Fuller, W. *Introduction to Statistical Time Series.* New York: John Wiley & Sons, 1996.

Gilbert, E. Pioneer maps of health and disease in England. *Geogr. J.* 124:172–183, 1958.

Golden Software Inc. *SURFER for Windows User's Guide.* Golden, CO: Golden Software Inc., 1994.

Gosh, M. Constrained Bayes estimation with applications. *J. Am. Stat. Assoc.* 87:533–540, 1992.

Greenland, S. Divergent biases in ecologic and individual-level studies. *Stat. Med.* 11:1209–1223, 1992.

Hahn, R. A., and D. F. Stroup. Race and ethnicity in public health surveillance: criteria for the scientific use of social categories. *Public Health Rep.* 109(1):7–15, 1994.

Haining, R. *Spatial Data Analysis in the Social and Environmental Sciences.* Cambridge: Cambridge University Press, 1990.

Hansen, K. Headbanging: robust smoothing in the plane. *IEEE Trans. Geosci. Remote Sensing* 29:369–378, 1991.

Kaluzny, S., S. Vega, T. Cardoso, and A. Shelly. *S + SPATIALSTATS User's Manual Version 1.0.* Seattle, WA: MathSoft, Inc., 1996.

Kass, R., and D. Steffey. Approximate bayesian inference in conditionally independent hierarchical models (parametric empirical Bayes models). *J. Am. Stat. Assoc.* 84:717–726, 1989.

Klaucke, D. N. Evaluating public health surveillance. In: *Principles and Practices of Public Health Surveillance,* edited by S. M. Teutsch, and E. Churchill. New York: Oxford University Press, 1994.

Laird, N., and T. A. Louis. Empirical Bayes confidence intervals based on bootstrap samples. *J. Am. Stat. Assoc.* 82:739–750, 1987.

Louis, T. A. Estimating a population of parameter values using Bayes and empirical Bayes methods. *J. Am. Stat. Assoc.* 79:393–398, 1984.

Louis, T. A. Using empirical Bayes methods in biopharmaceutical research. *Stat. Med.* 10:811–827, 1991.

Marshall, R. Mapping disease and mortality rates using empirical Bayes estimators. *Stat. Med.* 40:283–294, 1991a.

Marshall, R. A review of methods for the statistical analysis of spatial patterns of disease. *J. R. Stat. Soc.* 154:421–441, 1991b.

MathSoft. *S-PLUS Guide to Statistical and Mathematical Analysis.* Seattle, WA: MathSoft Inc., 1995.

Mollie, A. Bayesian mapping of disease. In: *Markov Chain Monte Carlo in Practice,* edited by W. Gilks, S. Richardson, and D. Spiegelhalter. New York: Chapman & Hall, 1996, pp. 359–379.

Mollie, A., and S. Richardson. Empirical Bayes estimates of cancer mortality rates using spatial models. *Stat. Med.* 10:95–112, 1991.

Pickle, L., W. Mason, N. Howard, R. Hoover, and J. Fraumeni. *Atlas of Cancer Morality Among Whites, 1950–1980.* Washington, DC: U.S. Government Printing Office, DHHS Publication No. 87–2900, 1987.

Radiological Assessments Corporation. *Draft Report, Task 6: Radiation Doses and Risks to Residents from FMPC Operations from 1951–1988,* Vol. I. Atlanta: Centers for Disease Control and Prevention, 1996.

Rothman, K. J. A sobering start for the cluster busters' conference. *Am. J. Epidemiol.* 132:S6–S13, 1990.

Shopland, D., A. Hartman, J. Gibson, M. Mueller, L. Kessler, and W. Lynn. Cigarette smoking among U.S. adults by state and region: estimates from the current population survey. *J. Nat. Cancer Inst.* 88:1748–1758, 1996.

Singh, A., and G. Roberts. State space modeling of cross classified time series of counts. *Int. Stat. Rev.* 60:321–335, 1992.

Stone, R. Investigations of excess environmental risks around putative sources: statistical problems and a proposed test. *Stat. Med.* 7:649–660, 1988.

Thacker, S. B. Historical development. In: *Principles and Practices of Public Health Surveillance,* edited by S. M. Teutsch and E. Churchill. New York: Oxford University Press, 1994.

Thacker, S. B., D. F. Stroup, and R. G. Parrish. Public health surveillance in environmental health. *Am. J. Public Health* 86:633–638, 1996.

Tukey, J. *Exploratory Data Analysis.* Reading, PA: Addison-Wesley, 1977.

Tukey, P., and J. Tukey. Graphical display of data sets in 3 or more dimensions. In: *Interpreting Multivariate Data,* edited by V. Barnett. New York: John Wiley & Sons, 1981.

Waller, L., B. Carlin, H. Xia, and A. Gelfand. Hierarchical spatio-temporal mapping of disease rates. *J. Am. Stat. Assoc.* 92:607–617, 1997.

Waller, L., and G. Jacquez. Disease models implicit in statistical tests of disease clustering. *Epidemiology* 6:584–590, 1995.

Waller, L., and R. McMaster. *Geographic Information Systems and Public Health Surveillance.* Minneapolis: University of Minnesota, School of Public Health, Division of Biostatistics, Research Report 96–002, 1996.

Williamson, G. D., J. T. Massey, H. B. Schulman, S. Siebu, and S. T. Smith (Eds.). Symposium on quantitative methods for utilization of multi-source data in public health. *Stat. Med.* 14:516–517, 1995.

Zeger, S. A regression model for time series of counts. *Biometrika* 75:621–629, 1988.

5

Investigating Health Effects and Hazards in the Community

KAREN KAFADAR
JOHN S. ANDREWS, JR.

Members of a community often do not think about public health functions until an adverse health effect or hazard is suspected. When an outbreak arises due to a communicable disease; a technological or manmade disaster; an environmental toxin; or contaminated food, water, or air, a community can quickly mobilize itself for action. Frequently, the local public health authority is responsible for taking such action. However, if the problem continues or has been inadequately addressed, a community may solicit help from state and federal agencies. The local health authority must address these concerns quickly, forthrightly, and completely to maintain its credibility.

The first priority of public health personnel is to reduce mortality and morbidity. Adverse health effects must be treated, and continued exposure to the hazardous substance or new illness must be prevented. Therefore, the first activities to occur after identifying an adverse health effect or hazard in the community are to provide medical treatment to ill persons and to interrupt ongoing exposure (e.g., providing emergency medical treatment for injured persons, evacuating persons from their homes or businesses, or having the gas and electric utility companies temporarily discontinue services).

In many areas of the world, medical care systems are excellent, so public health personnel may not be involved in the actual treatment of ill persons. However, their authority may be helpful in obtaining police assistance to control traffic; organizing various parts of the medical care system to work together; and obtaining laboratory testing for food-, water-, or airborne contaminants.

Some questions can be used to quickly identify a point of contact and to characterize a situation: What is the name of the caller? What is the caller's role or position in the current event? How can I contact the caller again? What does the caller suspect the problem is? Does the problem appear to be the cause of illness or death? How many persons have died? (This question actually combines two questions, Has anyone died? and How many?) How many have been sent to hospitals? How many others are ill? What are the signs and symptoms of ill persons? When did the first person become ill? How much time elapsed between the event that caused the illness and the time the first person became ill? Are all ill persons being treated? What control measures have been instituted to prevent further illness? Should community leaders, the media, or any other persons be notified? What other information might be important to know?

Hypothesis Generation

From a public health viewpoint, the following steps are used to generate hypotheses about the cause of an adverse health effect or hazard in the community: *(1)* determine that a problem actually exists; *(2)* confirm the diagnosis for ill persons; *(3)* determine the characteristics that define a case and then count the number of cases; *(4)* obtain basic epidemiological and demographic information on the cases, including affected persons (age, gender, race), time (of exposure, of illness onset), place (of exposure, at time of illness, of concurrent activities); *(5)* determine who else is at risk of having the characteristics of a case; *(6)* develop and test a hypothesis for what caused persons to become exposed or ill; *(7)* compare the hypothesis with the epidemiological facts that are obtained; *(8)* develop and evaluate control measures; and *(9)* prepare a report and plan a systematic study.

After talking to several persons who are affected by the health effect or hazard, investigators quickly gain an idea of the problem, its scope, and some potential causes worth investigating. Investigators can determine whether the signs and symptoms are consistent with person-to-person spread of an infectious disease, eating a particular meal, drinking water from a specific source, breathing air in a particular location, being near a specific technological or natural hazard, or contacting a specific hazardous substance. After having collected and classified this information on person, time, and place, a hypothesis can be generated.

Statistical issues arise at several stages of the investigation. The treatment of ill persons requires accurate diagnostic procedures that are both *sensitive* to the detection of disease and *specific* to the disease or condition that caused the outbreak. Data collection for ill persons must be accurate, timely, and unbiased. The statistical hypothesis determines the design of the investigation, data from which will either confirm or refute it. Finally, conclusions based on the statistical investigation, including risk to the affected population, must be communicated in an interpretable fashion.

Examples

Misdiagnosis of Guillain-Barré Syndrome

In the spring of 1982, a health officer in Jamaica called the Caribbean Epidemiology Centre (CAREC) in Port-of-Spain, Trinidad, to report an epidemic of Guillain-Barré syndrome. Illness had occurred among children throughout the island during the previous weeks. According to the health officer, the occurrence of these cases of Guillain-Barré was unusual and problematic, especially in view of the fact that no changes had occurred in their ongoing vaccination programs.

CAREC staff knew that no similar outbreaks had occurred in 17 other English-speaking Caribbean countries that reported illness to CAREC (see Chapter 4 for a discussion of surveillance). They noted that all cases of illness involved children; Guillain-Barré would be expected to occur in adults as well. By monitoring health indicators throughout the Caribbean over several previous years, CAREC also knew that polio immunization rates in Jamaica had been decreasing and that electricity production had been sporadic as a result of limited financial resources. Even if vaccine were available, it may not have been kept sufficiently cool to maintain its potency.

These data regarding persons (i.e., children), time (i.e., spring season), and place (i.e., Jamaica, having modest financial and public health resources), obtained from one telephone call and combined with knowledge of the public health situation in Jamaica, cast doubt on the hypothesis of Guillain-Barré syndrome as the illness and suggested instead poliomyelitis. Answers to certain epidemiological questions suggested the hypothesis, later confirmed by a community investigation.

Typhoid Fever Outbreak

In 1980, after Hurricane Allen in Jamaica, several persons in one community were diagnosed by their physicians as having typhoid fever on the basis of clinical signs and symptoms. Public health personnel were asked to investigate the outbreak. Data regarding persons, time, and place again were collected. All persons who were ill came from one specific area of the island (persons); citizens reported that, after the hurricane (time), a tree had fallen and broken a pipe that brought water from the top of a nearby hill (place) to provide the community water supply. Citizens on both sides of a ravine had to find alternate sources of water. A map of the typhoid fever victims showed that illness occurred only among persons who lived on one side of the ravine; no illness was observed among those who lived on the other side.

From this information, public health officials developed the hypothesis that water sources serving persons on each side of the ravine were different. A case-control investigation (using the steps listed in the section Confirming a Hypothesis, below) confirmed typhoid fever. Citizens living on the side of the ravine with the contaminated water source were interviewed and reported getting water from a "spring" after the pipe was broken. A visit to the "spring" revealed a small pool of water, likely the source of the typhoid organisms.

Confirming a Hypothesis

Once the hypothesis for the cause of the outbreak is determined, it must be confirmed with a valid study. Although no study can ever be 100% conclusive, a study can be designed to have a high probability of confirming the hypothesis if, in fact, it is correct. This section will describe possible study designs and focus on one of the most common for investigating community outbreaks, the case-control study.

Types of Studies

Studies can be divided into the following three types that describe their purpose: descriptive, analytic, and experimental. Descriptive studies aim to collect information about signs, symptoms, times, places, and persons affected by the outbreak; as such, they are useful in generating hypotheses. To confirm or deny a hypothesis, analytic or experimental studies must be conducted.

Experimental Studies

In *experimental studies*, the investigator can affect events by administering some treatment or intervention to a group of persons to evaluate the effects of such intervention. The most convincing experimental study design is the *randomized controlled trial*, where subjects are randomized into two or more groups (e.g., exposed or not exposed to the hazard) (Byar, 1988). After a preestablished length of time, the numbers of cases of illness in the different groups are compared. When subjects are truly randomized among groups, possible risk factors for subjects should be balanced across the groups, so the different numbers of cases in the groups will stem from either statistical variation or the exposure—and if the difference is too large to be ascribed to statistical variation, the only remaining explanation is exposure. This type of trial was conducted in the 1954 field trial of the Salk poliomyelitis vaccine: subjects were either exposed or not exposed to the vaccine, and the numbers of polio cases that developed in the two groups were compared (Meier, 1989). The potential for bias with this type of study is very low. Unfortunately, for ethical reasons, this type of study often cannot be conducted: subjects cannot be randomized to a group that is already suspected of being harmful, such as exposure to chemicals.

Analytic Studies

When the investigator merely records events rather than influencing their outcome through a treatment or intervention, the study is called *analytic* or *descriptive*. Examples of analytic studies are different types of *cohort studies* and the *case-control study*.

With the *prospective cohort study*, participants with varying levels of exposure to the hazard are identified in advance, data on risk factors are collected, and then cases develop as the study progresses. The dates, times, and amounts of exposure received by each person are noted over time. Because information can be collected in advance, procedures for determining exposure and disease outcome are more consistent and reliable. Moreover, several disease outcomes can be identified, and trends in increased levels of exposure (e.g., to radiation, asbestos, or passive smoke) can be estimated. Depending on the disease, a sufficient number of cases may occur in minutes (e.g., acute environmental hazards), days or weeks (e.g., infectious diseases), or years (e.g., environmental hazards); thus, because this type of study must wait for cases to develop, it is feasible only when the incubation period is very short, or when results are not expected for several years and resources are available for prolonged study (e.g., the Framingham Heart Study and the Baltimore Longitudinal Aging Study). Once enough cases of disease have occurred, investigators analyze the results and determine whether exposure was associated with the particular element or chemical under investigation. The main advantage of these studies is that information is obtained on everyone before exposure has occurred, so the two groups of persons, exposed and not exposed, are likely to be homogeneous in terms of other environmental conditions. The main disadvantage of these types of studies is that years or decades may elapse before enough cases of disease have been diagnosed—and the power of a study depends on the number of cases (see Chapter 2 and the section Matched Controls, later in this chapter).

To avoid the potentially long wait for cases to develop, the *retrospective cohort study* uses records and interviews to determine past exposure status of a study participant, and then follows the medical history of the subject over time to see whether and when disease develops. As in the prospective cohort study, the participant is initially free of disease. Risk factors, exposure status, and health outcome are assessed at different times. In contrast, the *cross-sectional cohort study* determines both the covariates and the outcome at the same time. These types of studies are appropriate when the covariates (e.g., exposure status or other risk factors) do not change over time or by the outcome (either illness or health). For example, the cross-sectional cohort study would not be suitable for a study of smoking and lung cancer, because development of any sort of cancer might encourage the study participant to quit smoking—and thus smoking status would change over the duration of the study.

With community hazards, cases have often already appeared, and the urgency of most outbreaks requires that a study be designed and conducted expeditiously and efficiently. In other situations, the risk may cause disease that is either relatively uncommon or is very slow to develop. For both reasons—urgency and low incidence—a *case-control study* is appropriate. Here, study participants are classified retrospectively on the basis of disease outcome, with present ("case") or absent ("control"). In fact, controls can (and should) be chosen to match characteristics unrelated to the disease outcome among the cases. The subjects are then further cross-classified according to their exposure status, and the proportion of cases among those exposed is compared with that among those who were not exposed.

Case-Control Studies

Case-control studies are extremely useful for investigating outbreaks in a community, especially when the disease is rare, when the time between exposure and disease is long, and when results are needed quickly. The investigator must develop a comprehensive questionnaire from which association can be assessed and data can be analyzed quickly. This type of study raised the initial suspicions about increased risk of lung cancer as the result of tobacco exposure, because the time between exposure and development of disease takes 20 years or more (Doll and Hill, 1964a,b). Moreover, participants cannot be randomized to a smoking group, so experimental studies are not appropriate. Prospective cohort studies have confirmed the results of case-control studies showing an association between tobacco exposure and lung cancer. Because cases are highly overrepresented in the study population compared with a typical population, the rates of outcomes within exposure categories cannot be estimated as they can be with a prospective cohort study, but a case-control study can be designed to give accurate assessments of association between disease and exposure.

Designing a Case-Control Study

In November 1996, several cases of *Escherichia coli* bacterial infection occurred in the United States, primarily in western states. Eventually the cause was traced to an organic fruit juice company. How was this cause ascertained? How was the hypothesis generated, and how was it later confirmed? Because urgency was a critical factor, a case-control study had to be conducted quickly. The steps in designing a good case-control study are given in the following section. Many of these steps also apply to randomized control and prospective cohort study designs.

Literature Review

Previous studies may provide information related to the hypothesis of interest and guidance on the design of a new study. For example, certain causes may be more likely for some sorts of outbreaks, and certain confounders (e.g., disease comorbidity or age) may suggest factors on which controls should be matched to cases to reduce variability among case-control pairs. Other biases in earlier studies may be noted with specific efforts to avoid them (e.g., expanded populations to reduce selection bias or improved survey design to reduce errors in misclassification or recall).

Matched Controls

Identification of suspected causes cannot be made by interviewing only affected persons; for comparison, healthy persons (controls) also must be interviewed. In situations where a nationally distributed food-borne contaminant is suspected, both case patients and controls must be surveyed for their food intake in the days and hours leading up to the outbreak. The idea behind matching controls to cases is to remove any other possible explanation except the exposure of interest for the increased rate of disease among exposed versus nonexposed persons. If controls are similar to cases in every way, except the presence of disease, then the difference in disease risk can be attributed only to exposure. An example of erroneous conclusions resulting from poorly matched groups is a study that tries to identify an association between hormone replacement therapy and breast cancer incidence: if all case patients had at least one breast cancer death among their immediate relatives and controls tended to have no deaths, it would be impossible to sort out whether any observed increased risk of disease was due to the genetic component or to hormone replacement therapy. One way to avoid such misattribution is to find controls who are similar to case patients in disease history, relatives' health, age, occupation, ethnicity, and socioeconomic status. Then, by designing a survey to prompt accurate recall and minimize sources of confounding (see section Collecting Data, below), a list of substances that might be involved can be isolated. For more detailed discussion of this topic, see Armitage and Berry (1993), Garb (1996), and Fisher and van Belle (1993).

Collecting Data

The first issue to consider in collecting data is the objective. One possible objective may be to assess the presence and level of exposure in both cases and controls with an aim toward identifying differences. Exposures should be identified by type, time, and source, if known. This information will help isolate the cause. An exposure to which all cases and no controls have been subjected is strong evidence for association and possibly cause of disease; conversely, an exposure to which both cases and controls have been exposed in roughly the same proportions is unlikely to be the cause. At what point between these two extremes is an exposure deemed to have a "statistically significant" probability of being a cause for the outbreak? Statistical evaluation of case-control studies is described in the Analysis section, later in this chapter.

Sample Size

How many case patients and controls are needed to identify a "statistically significant" elevated risk for disease? Clearly, a study of only three case patients and three controls, regardless of their exposure status, will be less convincing than one with 300 cases and 300 controls. The expected number of cases (each matched to one control) required to detect a significantly elevated risk in the presence of sampling variation depends on four quantities: *(1)* how high an increased risk is to be detected (e.g., a twofold or a fivefold increase); *(2)* the probability that the study will detect such an increase (e.g., a study that has only a 50% chance of being declared "significant" when the true relative risk is really 2.5 is equally likely to conclude either "no effect" or "statistically significant difference"—which may be too low to justify spending the resources); *(3)* the probability of asserting an elevated risk when in fact there is none (i.e., type I error); and *(4)* the proportion of controls who were exposed to the suspected hazard. Sample size requirements are described in Chapter 2 for general studies and in the section Statistical Considerations: Power in this chapter for case-control studies specifically.

Sources of Confounding

Case-control studies are always subject to more biases than are experimental and randomized trials or prospective cohort studies. Case-control participants are asked about their disease and exposure status, and their recall is likely not to be perfectly accurate ("recall bias"). Carefully conducted studies will confirm disease status with medical records, but exposure status is harder to confirm beyond the subject's word. Other sources of study bias involve confounding variables. For example, a case-control study might establish a link between smoking and cervical cancer—but only because women with certain sexual practices may be more likely to smoke; the real association with cervical cancer is sexual practice. Smoking is merely a confounder. Poorly matched controls can result in misattribution of association. Despite these limitations, the benefits of conducting a case-control study can outweigh the potential for bias, especially if steps are taken to minimize potential confounders as described in previous sections.

Discussion Questions

1. What various types of studies can be used to confirm or refute a hypothesis concerning a potential cause for illness in a community? What are the advantages and limitations of each?

2. To pose the question, How many subjects do I need to detect whether a hazard or environmental exposure is related to the occurrence of disease? Four quantities are needed. What are they? Can you provide intuitive explanations for why the sample size depends on these quantities?

Survey Design and Analysis

Information on cases may be available via hospital records and surveillance systems; controls should be selected to match cases as closely as possible. In this section, some issues are discussed that relate to obtaining data on these persons to help answer the primary question of interest.

Design: Validity and Efficiency

The measures of a good survey are its validity (i.e., obtaining correct information) and its efficiency (i.e., the precision with which information is obtained). When the survey is aimed at confirming the presence of a specific substance or exposure, the questionnaire can be focused and relatively straightforward. But when the substance is unknown, the survey questions must cover a broad range of possibilities, including typical exposures in daily living and a complete assessment of dietary intake. Because many of these items are likely to be so commonplace that persons are likely to overlook them, a good survey must be designed to encourage recollection of routine activities (e.g., drinking water and walking a pet in a park).

Invariably, costs must be taken into consideration in designing a survey. Written questionnaires are inexpensive; they are also subject to low response and consequently may be biased due to the lack of information from nonresponders (e.g., only the moderately ill may respond because healthy persons are not interested and the extremely ill are too ill to participate). For outbreaks, face-to-face interviews may be more cost effective, because more valuable information will be obtained than can be solicited in a questionnaire, particularly if an observant interviewer follows up on important replies. Sometimes questionnaires can be distributed en masse to a large segment of the population, case patients and controls (e.g., on a cruise ship or in a small community), and supplemented by a sampling of face-to-face interviews.

Two important considerations in designing surveys, coverage and length, are often at conflict. Without complete coverage, the cause can be missed entirely if the list of exposures fails to include the culprit. On the other hand, participants resent extensive surveys that take considerable time. The challenge is to design a survey or interview to accommodate both criteria. Another practical consideration is cost, especially with face-to-face interviews. If the interview is short, most of the cost involves travel time, and an efficient design will designate clusters of interviews in specific single areas. Telephone interviews can be nearly as effective as face-to-face interviews, particularly if potential participants are provided in advance with a written "crib sheet" of possible responses (e.g., "every day," "frequently," "sometimes," "rarely," "never").

Regardless of the type of survey, it is important to remember that survey results apply only to the population that was sampled and may not apply to other populations. The most common types of nonsampling errors in a survey arise from incomplete population coverage and nonresponse, both of which can cause biases in the results. By defining the extent of the outbreak and the likely targets for infection, and following up on nonresponders, both of these errors can be reduced. Finally, all surveys should be subjected to a pilot study to ensure relevance and unambiguity in the questions and to identify possible confounding in the replies.

Analysis

In discussing analysis we use the results from a study conducted to confirm a hypothesis, first by testing it, and then by examining statistical considerations and the design.

Testing the Generated Hypothesis

Suppose 100 patients who have *E. coli* infection and 100 matched controls are asked if they drank a particular brand of apple juice within the last 7 days, and the results are cross-tabulated as follows:

	Exposure		
	Yes (Drank)	No (Did Not Drink)	Total
Cases	95	5	100
Controls	5	95	100

These results leave little doubt about the association between apple juice consumption and disease. In fact, only about 25 tables could have provided more convincing evidence than the one above:

96	4
5	95

. . .
. . .

100	0
5	95

96	4
4	96

. . .
. . .

100	0
4	96

. . .
. . .

100	0
0	100

But what if the results had been less clear-cut, such as:

	Exposure		
	Yes (Drank)	No (Did Not Drink)	Total
Cases	60	40	100
Controls	45	55	100

How convincing is this evidence? Can the risk of disease from exposure be estimated? How much confidence do we have in our estimate of the risk? In this table, the risk for disease among those who drank can be estimated as 60/(60 + 45) = 0.5714, and, among those who did not, as 40/(40 + 55) = 0.4211. The ratio of estimated risks, called the *approximate relative risk*, is 0.5714/0.4211 = 1.357. That is, a person is 1.357 × more likely (35.7% higher risk) to have the disease after consuming this brand of apple juice. But suppose another case-control study is conducted, also with 200 persons, and the results are:

	Exposure		
	Yes (Drank)	No (Did Not Drink)	Total
Cases	54	46	100
Controls	40	60	100

Now the approximate relative risk is (54/95)(46/106) = 1.324, which is slightly lower. Statistical variation in the cell counts results in slightly different estimates.

If the true relative risk exceeds 1, then disease and exposure are related. A case-control study tries to estimate this risk. If the uncertainty in the estimate falls below 1, the association is not certain. An interval is needed that provides reasonable confidence (i.e., 95% confidence) of where the true relative risk lies. In the two previous tables, the 95% confidence intervals are (1.017, 1.810) and (1.002, 1.749). The lower endpoints of both intervals exceed 1 (although not by much), so marginal evidence exists of an association between exposure and disease.

The formulas for a general table are as follows:

Exposure

	Exposed	Not Exposed	Total
Cases	a	c	$(a+c)$
Controls	b	d	$(b+d)$
Total	$(a+b)$	$(c+d)$	

1. Estimate the relative risk, R, by $\hat{R} = [a/(a+b)]/[c/(c+d)]$. Let $T = \log_e \hat{R}$.
2. Calculate G, the uncertainty in T, given by the formula for the standard deviation (SD) of T: $G = SD(T) = [1/a - 1/(a+b) + 1/c - 1/(c+d)]^{1/2}$.
3. An approximate 95% confidence interval for the true relative risk, R, is $(\exp\{T - 1.96G\}, \exp\{T + 1.96G\})$.

These formulas were used to derive the confidence intervals for the two previous illustrations.

When the case is extremely rare, then a is small compared with b and c is small compared with d, so $\hat{R}$ is very close to the estimated *odds ratio*, $\hat{\phi}$, given by $\hat{\phi} = (ad)/(bc)$. The uncertainty in $t = \log_e \hat{\phi}$ is approximately $G = SD(t) = [1/a + 1/b + 1/c + 1/d]^{1/2}$, so an approximate 95% confidence interval for the true odds ratio ϕ is $(\exp\{t - 1.96G\}, \exp\{t + 1.96G\})$.

Statistical Considerations: Power

The above formulas can lend insight into the number of observed cases needed to establish an association between disease and exposure. The width of the confidence intervals involves the numbers in the four cells; the larger these numbers, the less uncertainty and the greater the likelihood of detecting a truly elevated risk in disease. For example, suppose a 20% increase in risk resulting from exposure is important enough to be detected. A study is designed to include 20 case patients, 12 (60%) of whom were exposed; and 20 controls, 6 (30%) of whom were exposed. Then, using the formulas for the estimated odds ratio and the uncertainty, $\hat{\phi} = (12 \cdot 14)/(6 \cdot 8) = 3.5$, $t = \ln\hat{\phi} = 1.253$, $G = SE(\hat{\phi}) = 0.668$, and an approximate 95% confidence interval is $\exp(1.253 \pm 1.96 \cdot 0.668) = (0.945, 12.975)$. Statistical significance is close at $p = 0.05$, but the values are not quite statistically significant (p-value is 0.06). If the study had included 60 case patients and 60 controls, again with 30% of controls exposed to the potential hazard, then

Exposure

	Yes	No	Total
Cases	$a = 36$	$c = 18$	$(a + c) = 54$
Controls	$b = 24$	$d = 42$	$(b + d) = 66$
Total	$(a + b) = 60$	$(c + d) = 60$	120

The odds ratio is still 3.5, but now $G = [1/36 + 1/24 + 1/18 + 1/42]^{1/2} = 0.3858$. A 95% confidence interval is

$$\exp\{\ln(3.5) \pm 1.96 \cdot 0.3858\} = \exp\{1.253 \pm 0.756\} = \exp\{0.497, 2.009\} = (1.644, 7.456)$$

Now the data are sufficient to suggest that indeed the true relative risk exceeds 1; in fact, the p-value is about 0.0012.

This illustration demonstrates the importance of conducting a study large enough that it has a high probability of detecting a truly elevated risk of disease resulting from exposure (i.e., high power; see Chapter 2). Table 5.1 provides the expected number of cases in a case-control study (with one matched control per case) required to produce an 80% chance of "statistical significance at $p = 0.05$" for given values of the odds ratio and the proportion of controls exposed to the hazard. A more complete table can be found in Armitage and Berry (1993, p. 580). The odds ratio has the greater influence on the sample size. Notice that usually 100 case patients and 100 controls are needed to have at least an 80% chance of finding an odds ratio of 2.5 "significant" ($p < 0.05$); even with such a large study, there is still a 20% chance of obtaining results that were split between exposed and unexposed in a way that could not achieve statistical significance (e.g., $a = 90$, $b = 10$, $c = 80$, $d = 20$). The numbers are more than 200 if the odds ratio is only 2. Thus, a community that has only 20 cases is unlikely to demonstrate a

Table 5.1 Number of Cases (and Equal Number of Controls) Needed to Detect a Significant ($p = 0.05$) Relative Risk (> 1), with 80% Power

Proportion of Exposed Controls	Odds Ratio						
	1.5	2	2.5	3	4	5	10
0.05	1775	560	301	200	117	82	34
0.10	958	307	168	113	68	48	22
0.20	562	187	105	72	45	34	17
0.30	447	153	88	62	40	31	18
0.40	407	144	85	61	41	32	20

"statistically significant" risk, unless the hazard poses a tenfold risk for disease. If the study does not have reasonably high power for detecting the size of increased risk deemed important, the resources spent in designing it may be better spent on community efforts to educate the public or to reduce the potential for exposure to the hazard altogether.

Analysis of Matched Pairs Designs

Usually our selection of controls matches the cases only in the aggregate (i.e., on average, characteristics like the average age, proportion of females, and percentage Hispanics are about the same in both groups). When individual cases are carefully matched with individual controls on a case-by-case basis rather than simply in the aggregate, either by designing a case-control study or by matching persons or households in a survey, a huge source of variability is eliminated, namely the variability within subjects or subject pairs themselves. The study is likely to have higher power to detect a significant association between disease and exposure by eliminating variability that can interfere with our assessments. The analog of the *matched pairs t-test* (see Chapter 2) in this situation is *McNemar's test*, because recorded outcomes for each person can be either 1 (exposed) or 0 (not exposed):

Pair	Case (x_i)	Control (y_i)	Difference (d_i)
1	1	0	1
2	0	0	0
3	0	1	−1
4	1	1	0
etc.			

Four possible combinations are shown as subject pairs 1, 2, 3, 4 above. For n pairs of data, let n_{00} (respectively, n_{11}) be the number of pairs for which both case and control were unexposed (respectively, exposed), and let n_{01} (respectively, n_{10}) be the number of pairs for which the case but not the control was unexposed (respectively, exposed). Then the data of ones and zeroes can be summarized by

		Control is	
		Not Exposed	Exposed
Case is	Not exposed	n_{00}	n_{01}
	Exposed	n_{10}	n_{11}

The formulas for the matched pairs t-test on these binary data of n pairs are:

$$\bar{x} = (n_{10} + n_{11})/n$$
$$\bar{y} = (n_{01} + n_{11})/n$$
$$\bar{d} = \bar{x} - \bar{y} = (n_{10} - n_{01})/n$$

$$s^2_{\bar{d}} = \sum_{i=1}^{n} (d_i - \bar{d})^2/[n(n-1)] = [(n_{01} + n_{10}) - (n_{10} - n_{01})^2/n]/[n(n-1)]$$

When n is very large, $(n_{10} - n_{01})^2/n \ll (n_{01} + n_{10})$ and $n(n-1) \approx n^2$, and so

$$t\text{-statistic} = \bar{d}/s_{\bar{d}} \approx (n_{10} - n_{01})/(n_{01} + n_{10})^{1/2}$$

Under the null hypothesis, this statistic should have a Student's t distribution on $n - 1$ degrees of freedom, or, because n is large, as a normal distribution, its square should have a chi-squared distribution on 1 degree of freedom. McNemar's statistic is simply the square of the t-statistic given above; hence it is compared to the quantiles of a chi-squared distribution of 1 degree of freedom.

To illustrate McNemar's test, suppose a study involves 100 case-control pairs, and each case is matched carefully with a control. Of these 100 pairs, suppose that both case patient and control were exposed in 5 pairs, neither was exposed in 50 pairs, cases but not the controls were exposed in 30 pairs, and controls but not the cases were exposed in 15 pairs. Then McNemar's statistic is $(30 - 15)^2/(30 + 15) = 5.0$, significant at $p = 0.025$.

Further Issues

Multiple Hypotheses

The investigation of an outbreak may suggest more than one exposure. In this section we address the statistical considerations involved in testing multiple hypotheses.

Statistical Significance

As explained in Chapter 2, a null hypothesis that is rejected at "$p < 0.05$" means that only a 5% chance exists that the study would have produced a test statistic more extreme from what would be expected if in fact the null hypothesis were true. Because such extreme values are not likely to occur, a more probable inference is that the null hypothesis ("no association between disease and exposure") is not likely true, and the alternative hypothesis ("an association exists between disease and exposure") is more likely. But such extreme values do occur, 5% of the time. The chance of winning the Colorado lottery by picking all 6 of 36 numbers is only 1 in 1,947,792—but when 2 million persons play the lottery twice a week, several persons will win over the course of time. Similarly, even if absolutely no association exists between exposure and disease, a 5% chance exists that a test statistic will be significant, and the existence of an association that does not exist will be wrongly asserted. Of course, if the study is conducted only once, then the more likely explanation is that the null hypothesis is false. But it is possible that 19 additional replications of this study would all fail to show significance.

Now suppose 100 substances are tested for association between exposure and disease and 100 test statistics are generated, 5 of which are "significant at $p < 0.05$." Based on the preceding argument, it should not be a surprise; by chance alone, $0.05 \times 100 = 5$ tests should be significant when no association exists between disease and any of the exposures. In fact, if no association exists between disease and exposure to and of K substances, a certain number is expected to be significant just by chance, namely $0.05 \times K \pm 0.36\sqrt{K}$. (This formula is based on a 90% confidence interval for the number of "successes" in a binomial random variable whose probability of "success" is 0.05.) For 100 hypotheses, as many as seven to nine test statistics can be "significant" by chance alone.

Bonferroni Correction

One way to avoid making too many false conclusions is to lower the significance level of the test statistic. For example, with 100 hypotheses, each individual p-value could be required to be less than 0.0005, so that, on average, no more than $0.0005 \times 100 = 0.05$ hypotheses will be significant by chance. This added stringency raises the chi-squared statistic on 1 degree of freedom from 3.842 to 12.117 to achieve statistical significance using McNemar's test (Fisher and Van Belle, 1993). This "Bonferroni correction to the significance level" accounts for multiple hypotheses; it is convenient, easy to use, and easy to remember, but it is conservative.

Controlling the False Discovery Rate

The Bonferroni correction controls the number of false significant tests, or the number of the K null hypotheses that are rejected erroneously. A different approach instead controls the *false discovery rate*, or the expected proportion of falsely rejected hypotheses. This criterion integrates both the number of falsely rejected hypotheses, and the probability of a false rejection, given that the hypothesis was rejected. To ensure that the expected proportion of rejected hypotheses does not exceed 5%, on average, one approach is:

1. Rank all hypotheses in order of their p-values, so the hypothesis with the smallest p-value has rank 1. Denote these values $p_{(1)}, p_{(2)}, \ldots, p_{(K)}$.
2. Compare each $p_{(i)}$ with $0.05 \cdot i/K$ starting with the largest p-value, $p_{(K)}$. Let I be the first value of i, $i = K, K-1, K-2, \ldots$, for which $p_{(i)} \leq 0.05 \cdot i/K$.
3. Reject all null hypotheses whose p-values fail to exceed $p_{(i)}$.

This procedure tends to be less conservative than the Bonferroni correction; the theory can be found in Benjamini and Hochberg (1993). As an illustration, suppose the p-values from $K = 10$ hypotheses are: {0.001, 0.002, 0.005, 0.010, 0.040, 0.120, 0.243, 0.350, 0.368, 0.800}. Starting with $K = 10$, $p_{(10)} = 0.800$ is not less than $0.05 \cdot K/K = 0.05$, and likewise with $K = 9, 8, \ldots, 5$. When $K = 4$, $p_{(4)} = 0.01$, less than $0.05 \cdot 4/K = 0.02$. Hence $I = 4$, and the four hypotheses corresponding to the four smallest p-values are rejected.

Regardless of which procedure is applied, the existence of multiple hypotheses must be noted, and significance levels should be adjusted accordingly.

Models for Multiple Measurements

When collecting data on persons to investigate causes of outbreaks, more than one piece of information, in addition to disease status (health or ill, case or control), on each person is often obtained: age, exposure status, preexisting conditions, and smoking status. Sometimes these *covariates* can be valuable in identifying factors of comorbidity or increased risk of disease. The following paragraphs discuss briefly some ways in which such multivariate data may be analyzed using statistical models.

Logistic Regression

Chapter 2 describes multiple linear regression, where a continuous outcome [e.g., the logarithm of incidence in acquired immunodeficiency syndrome (AIDS) in a state or county] is modeled as a linear function of several variables (e.g., the logarithm of the state or city population, the net migration rate into the city, percentage of the population classified as nonwhite):

$$\text{Outcome} = \beta_0 + \beta_1 \cdot x_1 + \beta_2 \cdot x_2 + \beta_3 \cdot x_3 + \text{Residual} \qquad [5\text{--}1]$$

where, for example, $x_1 = \log(\text{population})$, $x_2 = $ net migration rate, $x_3 = $ percentage nonwhite, all of which can take on a wide range of values.

For the types of studies discussed in this chapter, the outcome is often binary: 0 (healthy, or control), or 1 (ill, or case-patient). Equation [5–1] would not be a meaningful model, because a linear function of continuous-valued variables will be continuous—not binary-valued. Nonetheless, the idea of a linear combination of covariates is appealing because of its interpretability. So instead of modeling the 0-1 outcome directly, a function of the *probability* that the outcome equals one is modeled:

$$\text{logit}(p) = \ln\,[p/(1-p)] = \beta_0 + \beta_1 \cdot x_1 + \beta_2 \cdot x_2 + \beta_3 \cdot x_3 + \text{residual} \qquad [5\text{--}2]$$

where p is the probability of disease, or being ill, and $1 - p$ is the probability of being disease-free, or healthy. The coefficient of the variable x_i, β_i, turns out to be the logarithm of the odds ratio (cf. Chapter 2). Thus, not only is Equation [5–2] a more sensible model [logit(p) will be continuous-valued], but its coefficients are more interpretable.

These models allow the estimation of the likelihood of being ill, or of being a case patient versus a control, based on covariates such as age, smoking status, or previous history of disease. Thus, such models may confirm or rule out suspected hazards. For example, a community that exhibits a rather large number of lung cancer cases may not be so unusual if the data indicate that most lung cancer cases were among smokers, leaving very few cases to be explained by environmental "hazards." Many statistical packages fit models of the type using Equation [5–2] with various methods of estimation and return odds ratios and associate confidence intervals so that risks can be assessed [see Armitage and Berry (1993)].

Time-Series Data

The severity of an outbreak is often measured by the number of cases of a disease, compared with the numbers observed during previous weeks, periods, or months. A statistical comparison allows the assessment of whether the present observed number really is excessive in view of previous trends. Data that occur in time require specially tailored methods that account for their sequential nature.

Time-series data may be conveniently decomposed into four components: a long-term broadly varying trend, a seasonal component (e.g., monthly effects), cyclical variation (e.g., 5-year cycles), and irregular, or "residual," variation. If one or more periods exhibit counts of cases above and beyond what the model predicts for long-term, seasonal, and cyclical components (i.e., an unusually high residual), investigation may be warranted.

The most convenient approach to understanding such series is to proceed in stages. This approach can be illustrated by analyzing the numbers of cases of tuberculosis (TB) in 13 four-week segments in each year from 1980 to 1989 (130 segments) that were reported to the National Notifiable Diseases Surveillance

System at the Centers for Disease Control and Prevention. Figure 5.1*A* plots the series and shows a broadly declining trend in the number of cases over the 10 year period. Thus, a line is fitted to these data by ordinary least squares (cf. Chapter 2):

$$y_t = 2097.04 - 5.3 \cdot t + e_t^{(1)}, t - 0, 1, \ldots, 129 \qquad [5\text{--}3]$$

For simplicity, this line has been fitted to the equally spaced time points, 0, 1, . . . , 129, although the slope and intercept are more interpretable if we rewrite Equation [5–3] in terms of years and fractions of years:

$$y_t = 1714.55 - 76.5 \cdot (x_t - 85) + e_t^{(1)}, x_t = 80, 80.069, 80.138, \ldots, 89.981 \quad [5\text{--}4]$$

Equation [5–4] shows about 1714 cases in 1985, with about 76 (more, less) cases for each year (before, after) 1985. In Figure 5.1*B*, the residuals from Equation [5–3] are plotted, namely:

$$e_t^{(1)} = y_t - 2097.04 + 5.3 \cdot t, t = 0, 1, \ldots, 129 \qquad [5\text{--}5]$$

The next fit is a seasonal component determined by the 4 week segments. A close inspection of Figure 5.1*B* suggests that the first and second 4 week segments tend to be slightly lower, and the last segment somewhat higher, than the intervening segments. Thus, from all ten data points in segment 1, their median, $s_1 = -550.8$, is subtracted, and likewise for the remaining 13 segments ($s_j =$ –211.4, 16.0, 1.0, –9.3, 3.2, 47.6, 67.1, –28.6, 123.6, 4.9, –63.1, 298.1, for $j = 2$, . . . , 13). Figure 5.1*C* plots the resulting residuals:

$$e_t^{(2)} = y_t - 2097.04 + 5.3 \cdot t - s_{[t/13]+1}, t = 0, 1, \ldots, 129 \qquad [5\text{--}6]$$

where $[t/13] + 1$ represents the largest integer in $t/13$, plus 1. These residuals seem to indicate a cycle that repeats itself approximately twice throughout the 10 years. So a cyclical trend is fit to these residuals of the form

$$e_t^{(2)} \approx M + A \cdot cos\,(\omega t) + B \cdot sin\,(\omega t) \qquad [5\text{--}7]$$

A rough estimate of ω can be determined by noting that, with two cycles in the 130 data points, the period is roughly 65 points, so ω is roughly $2\pi/65 = 0.10$. Least squares estimates for M, A, and B, as functions of ω, are given in Bloomfield (1976) (see also Chapter 2); the value of ω that minimizes the sum of the squared residuals from the fit is then chosen. For these data, the fit, shown in Figure 5.1C, is

$$\begin{aligned} e_t^{(2)} &\approx 23.21 + 17.92 \cdot cos\,(0.0847t) + 105.78 \cdot sin\,(0.0847t) \\ &= 23.21 + 107.29 \cdot cos\,(0.0847t - 1.403) \end{aligned} \qquad [5\text{--}8]$$

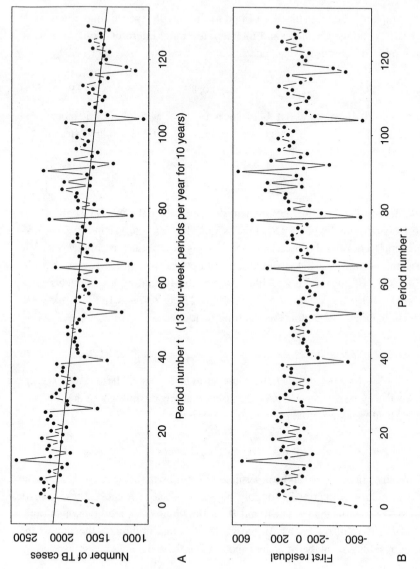

Figure 5.1. Tuberculosis cases, 1930–1939, United States. Period number ÷ (13 four-week periods per year for 10 years). *A*: Fitted line with intercept = 2128.9 and slope = ∇ − 5.432 *B*: Detrended data: first residual = number of cases − 2128.9 + 5.432 · *t*. *C*: Second residuals = first residuals with monthly readings averaged. *D*: Third residuals ... ...

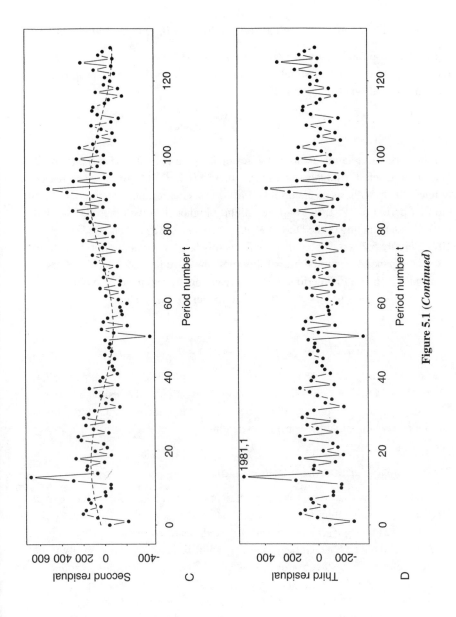

Figure 5.1 (*Continued*)

Interestingly, this frequency corresponds to a period of $2\pi/0.0847 = 74$, or roughly 5.7 years. Lastly, the final residuals are examined (Fig. 5.1D), accounting for all three terms: long-term, seasonal, and cyclical:

$$e_t^{(3)} = y_t - 2097.04 + 5.3 \cdot t - s_{[t/13]+1}$$
$$- 23.21 - 107.29 \cdot \cos(0.0847t - 1.403), t = 0, 1, \ldots, 129 \qquad [5\text{--}9]$$

Ideally, these final residuals are uncorrelated and have no structure. A statistic for testing the presence of serial correlation in these residuals was proposed by Durbin and Watson (1950, 1951):

$$d = \sum_{t=2}^{n} (e_t - e_{t-1})^2 / \sum_{t=1}^{n} (e_t - \bar{e})^2$$

If no serial correlation exists in the residuals, then the value of d should be 2. For the third set of residuals shown in Figure 5.1D, $d = 2.14$, giving us no reason to reject the hypothesis of uncorrelated residuals. One residual, corresponding to the first period of 1981, does appear slightly higher than the others (558). [For further understanding of the Durbin-Watson statistic, see Stuart and Ord (1991) p. 1077.] Figure 5.2 is a display that confirms this lack of correlation in the residuals, where panel A, a normal probability plot, shows rather nicely behaved residuals, apart from the first period of 1981 already noted, and panel B, a plot of $e_t^{(3)}$ versus $e_{t-1}^{(3)}$, shows no structure. The final model for these data is:

$$y_t \approx 2120.25 - 5.3 \cdot t + s_{[t/13]+1}$$
$$+ 107.29 \cdot \cos (0.0847t - 1.403), t = 0, 1, \ldots, 129 \qquad [5\text{--}10]$$

where $\{s_j, j = 1, \ldots, 13\} = \{-550.8, -211.4, 16.0, 1.0, -9.3, 3.2, 47.6, 67.1, -28.6, 123.6, 4.9, -63.1, 298.1\}$. The standard deviation of the residuals is about 115, so observations whose residuals deviate by more than roughly three times this value, or 345, might be worth investigating.

Longitudinal (Repeated Measures) Data

Sometimes multivariate data for a case patient or control are collected at several time points, thus combining multivariate data and time-series data. Usually the latter involves a single series of dozens or hundreds of observations. In contrast, longitudinal data are characterized by many short series (e.g., perhaps only three to ten time points measures for each person). Longitudinal data can be collected either retrospectively (e.g., "Did you have a disease/cigarette/exposure six months ago? Twelve months ago? Two years ago?") or prospectively, by following case patients and controls forward in time. Often, linear models are fit to these data as a function of the values of covariates, both present and past, but the methods of fitting must take into account the possible serial correlation of observations

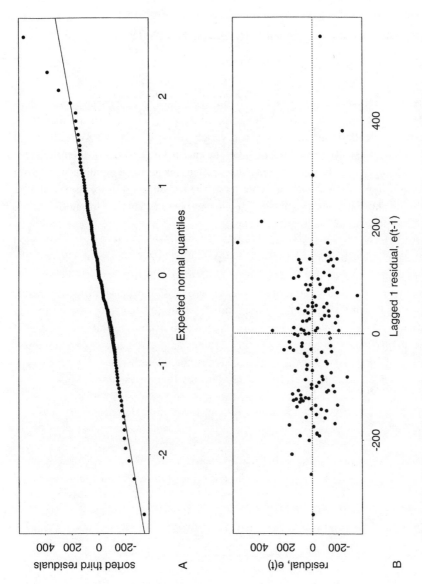

Figure 5.2. Demonstration confirming lack of correlation in the residuals of time-series data. *A*: Straight line indicates approximately normally distributed data. *B*: Lag-1 plot in third residuals.

in time on one person. These types of data are sometimes referred to as repeated measures data; two recent references for these types of models are Jones (1993) and Diggle (1998). Nonlinear longitudinal models are described in Davidian and Giltinan (1995).

Special Issues for Environmental Hazards

Similarity of Symptoms

The signs and symptoms of many infectious diseases (e.g., measles) are so characteristic that a simple physical examination often will confirm the diagnosis. Even for infectious agents that cause a variety of symptoms, the constellation of symptoms is usually similar enough that the causative agent can be identified easily. However, environmental exposures often result in symptoms that differ greatly from person to person. After exposure to benzene, for example, chronic lymphocytic leukemia might develop in one person, whereas in another acute myelogenous leukemia might develop.

Adverse health effects from exposure to environmental hazards can be very similar to adverse health effects being experienced by unexposed members of the community. For example, the background lifetime incidence rate of cancer is approximately 25% (i.e., about one in four persons will develop some sort of cancer during a lifetime). Thus, in a community of 1 million persons, approximately 250,000 cancers of various types are expected to occur over all age groups. If community members have been exposed to a hazard that causes 1 case of cancer in 1 million persons over a lifetime, identifying 1 extra case of cancer in the 250,000 that are expected to occur would be nearly impossible.

Dose

Because infectious agents multiply, the intensity of the exposure is usually not a major determinant of who becomes ill. However, with environmental exposures, the intensity and duration of exposure may make the difference between having acute symptoms, chronic symptoms, or no symptoms. Depending on the duration and intensity of exposure (dose), asbestos exposure might be the cause of only 1 or 2 cases of mesothelioma out of 100 persons who were exposed.

Latency

With infectious disease outbreaks, persons are likely to become ill within a few days or weeks. (Obvious exceptions include tuberculosis, leprosy, kuru, and human immunodeficiency virus, which may take months or years to develop.) With environmental exposures, illness may not occur for decades. For example, after exposure to benzene, cancer cases might not occur for 10 or more years. Similarly, mesothelioma might result from exposure to asbestos, but perhaps not for 20 years—and this condition may affect only a limited number of persons.

Memory

Adverse health effects from exposure have a long latency period. Persons may have great difficulty remembering what exposures they had 10 or 20 years earlier. By the time illness occurs, persons who were exposed may have moved to a different city, county, or state. Thus, even if a case of cancer is thought to have arisen from exposure to a specific environmental hazard, identifying where that exposure occurred may be difficult.

Lack of Information and Incomplete Understanding of Disease Process

The understanding of how environmental exposures cause disease is incomplete. Only recently has the technology been available to measure exposure to waterborne or airborne hazards. Monitors have been developed for occupational settings and now are being used in communities. Many communities, however, do not have measurements of the chemicals that were in their water or air 10 or 20 years ago.

Expense of Investigations

The expense of culturing an infectious agent is relatively minor compared with the expense of carrying out environmental monitoring for months or years. Thus, even when the technology is available, most communities do not have the resources to monitor their air, water, or soil for contaminants.

Political and Economic Considerations

Nearly everyone in a community will want to identify and eliminate hazards associated with adverse health effects. A community often will support efforts to obtain needed information on the signs, symptoms, age, sex, and concurrent activities of persons who are suspected cases. Likewise, communities often will co-operate to ensure that reliable information is obtained from well persons who had exposures similar to those ill persons.

However, when a hazard is a community environmental exposure, various community members may have differing views on whether adverse health effects occur as a result of exposure. If cases of disease have not occurred, even more controversy arises about whether a particular chemical really constitutes a community hazard. Often, companies connected with particular environmental hazards are major employers that are powerful in local, state, or national organizations.

Authorities are reluctant to impose sanctions on major employers for fear of endangering the economic welfare of these communities. As a result, confrontations may arise between local residents and local health authorities. Even when an investigation into a particular hazard has been initiated, local residents may complain about the pace of the investigation, and local health authorities may argue that excessive resources (staff time and money) have been spent on an issue that is not even confirmed to be a problem. Investigators of adverse health effects or a community hazard should be aware of the political and economic issues in the community.

Risk Communication

Risk communication is a complex, multidisciplinary, multidimensional, and evolving process of increasing importance for protecting the public's health. Public health officials communicate notions of risk to give citizens necessary and appropriate information and to involve them in making decisions that affect them. The public may not be readily familiar with the technology or statistical issues involved and so often has difficulty understanding them. Moreover, these complex issues frequently are surrounded by political controversy. A monograph that discusses health risk communication principles and practices has been written by Lum and Tinker (1994).

According to the National Research Council, "Risk communication is an interactive process of exchange of information and opinion among individuals, groups, and institutions. It involves multiple messages about the nature of risk and other messages, not strictly about risk, that express concerns, opinions, or reactions to risk messages or to legal and institutional arrangements for risk management" (National Research Council, 1989, p. 21). Risk communication is considered to be successful "to the extent that it raises the level of understanding of relevant issues or actions and satisfies those involved that they are adequately informed within the limits of available knowledge" (National Research Council, 1989, p. 26).

The U.S. Environmental Protection Agency (Covello and Allen, 1988) has identified "Seven Cardinal Rules of Risk Communication":

1. Accept and involve the public as a partner.
2. Plan carefully and evaluate your efforts.
3. Listen to the public's specific concerns.
4. Be honest, frank, and open.
5. Work with other credible sources.
6. Meet the needs of the media.
7. Speak clearly and with compassion.

Fischoff et al. (1981) identified factors that influenced risk perception:

Risks Perceived as Acceptable	Risks Perceived as Unacceptable
Voluntary	Imposed
Controlled by the individual	Controlled by others
Have clear benefits	Have little or no benefit
Distributed fairly	Distributed unfairly
Natural	Manmade
Statistical	Catastrophic
Generated by a trusted source	Generated by an untrusted source
Familiar	Exotic
Affect adults	Affect children

Community Empowerment

Issues of community empowerment rarely are important with infectious diseases, because infectious diseases most often do not have a political action community. These issues are very important, however, when adverse health effects are thought to be caused by environmental hazards.

In the past, the state or federal government usually enters the community, conducts an investigation, and then recommends specific actions. Because of political and economic issues (see previous section), communities want to be involved not only with the actions recommended but also with the investigation itself. Several models have been tried for involving the community, the most constructive and successful of which are Community Assistance Panels of the Agency for Toxic Substances and Disease Registry (ATSDR) and Technical Assistance Grants provided by the Environmental Protection Agency. Community participation is vital to successful investigations of adverse health effects and hazards because it increases chances of their acceptance and approval. This goal is accomplished most easily by involving community leaders early in the investigation and by making the process as open as possible. Including community members, both scientists and nonscientists, at the table with local, state, and federal health authorities, is important as is disseminating information early and frequently through newsletters, educational material, and community briefings.

Statistical Issues

The main statistical issue that is relevant to hypothesis generation is whether enough persons are exposed or ill to conduct an investigation that will confirm an association between an adverse health outcome and an exposure, if indeed such an association really exists. This is called the power of a study (see Chapter 2). For example, benzene exposure may really cause leukemia, but the one or two cases in a community of 300,000 persons are not enough to confirm this statistically.

The power of a study is related directly to the observed number of cases of illness. With adverse health effects in a community, many instances of disease may be caused by the person-to-person spread of a communicable disease; a food-, water-, or airborne illness; or a technological or manmade disaster. But very few cases of the suspected disease may occur, making it difficult to associate an exposure with, for example, a cluster of brain cancer, leukemia, or decreased IQ in children.

An additional problem is often the absence of quantitative measures of exposure, either because no one tried to measure exposure 5, 10, or 20 years ago when it occurred, or because exposure was so fleeting that, by the time a decision was made to measure it, it had already ended (e.g., radiation or certain chemicals), or because the testing equipment was too insensitive to measure low levels of exposure.

These issues raise an important question: Under what circumstances is it worthwhile to investigate an association between adverse health effects and exposures? Health studies can be very costly, especially if they are unlikely to have enough power to identify health effects.

Concern from the community and media may be so strong that a study must be conducted. In such cases, it is essential to make the objectives of the study and the magnitude of the risk that can be detected very clear. Resources may be available to ascertain, for example, a tenfold increase in cancer, but not a fivefold or twofold increase (i.e., a study conducted in a community where only a twofold increase in risk occurs may have only a very small probability of being "statistically" significant).

If a twofold increase is deemed important, then either more resources must be allocated or all parties involved must be content with the small probability that the study will detect such a low increase in risk.

Occasionally a study with relatively low power can be combined with other small studies in a meta-analysis. Issues in the design of a study to be used in connection with a meta-analysis involve comparability of studies and extensive literature reviews. Generally, a study should be planned so that its results can stand on the merits of its design.

A previous study of disease and its possible association with past exposures may not help to explain the current exposure situation. Because of many changes in the production and distribution of hazards over the past 20 years, situations that were common two decades ago are very different from today's situations.

References

Armitage, P., and G. Berry. *Statistical Methods in Medical Research*, 3rd ed. Oxford: Blackwell Scientific Publications, 1993.

Benjamini, Y., and Y. Hochberg. Controlling the false discovery rate: a practical and powerful approach to multiple testing. *J. R. Stat. Soc. [B]* 57(1):289–300, 1993.

Bloomfield, P. *Fourier Analysis of Time Series: An Introduction*. New York: John Wiley & Sons, 1976.

Byar, D. P. The use of data bases and historical controls in treatment comparisons. In: *Recent Results in Cancer Research, Vol. III: Cancer Clinical Trials: A Critical Appraisal*, edited by H. Scheurlen, and R. Kay. New York: Springer-Verlag, 1988, pp. 95–98.

Covello, V. and F. Allen. *Seven Cardinal Rules of Risk Communication*. Washington, DC: U.S. Environmental Protection Agency, Office of Policy Analysis, 1988.

Davidian, M., and D. Giltinan. *Nonlinear Models for Repeated Measurement Data*. London: Chapman & Hall, 1995.

Diggle, P. An approach to the analysis of repeated measurements. *Biometrics* 44:959–971, 1988.

Doll, R., and A. B. Hill. Mortality in relation to smoking: ten years' observations of British doctors. *Br. Med. J.* i:1399–1410, 1964a.

Doll, R., and A. B. Hill. Mortality in relation to smoking: ten years' observations of British doctors. *Br. Med. J.* i:1460–1467, 1964b.

Durbin, J., and G. S. Watson. Testing for serial correlation in least squares regression, I. *Biometrika* 37:409, 1950.

Durbin, J., and G. S. Watson. Testing for serial correlation in least squares regression, II. *Biometrika* 38:159, 1951.

Fischhoff, B., S. Lichtenstein, P. Slovic, and D. Kenney. *Acceptable Risk*. Cambridge, MA: Cambridge University Press, 1981.

Fisher, L. D., and G. van Belle. *Biostatistics: A Methodology for the Health Sciences*. New York: John Wiley & Sons, 1993.

Garb, J. L. *Understanding Medical Research: A Practitioner's Guide*. Boston: Little, Brown & Co., 1996.

Jones, R. H. *Longitudinal Data with Serial Correlation: A State-Space Approach*. New York: Chapman & Hall, 1993.

Lum, M. R., and T. L. Tinker. *A Primer on Health Risk Communication Principles and Practices*. Atlanta, GA: Agency for Toxic Substances and Disease Registry, Public Health Service, U.S. Department of Health and Human Services, 1984.

Meier, P. The biggest public health experiment ever: the 1954 field trial of the Salk poliomyelitis vaccine. *Statistics: A Guide to the Unknown.* Belmont, CA: Wadsworth, 1989, pp. 3–14.

National Research Council. *Improving Risk Communication.* Washington, DC: Committee on Risk Perception and Communication, National Academy Press, 1989, p. 21.

Stuart, A., and J. K. Ord. *Kendall's Advanced Theory of Statistics*, Vol. 2, 5th ed. New York: Oxford University Press, 1991.

6

Setting Priorities for Health Needs and Managing Resources

MARTIN MELTZER
STEVEN M. TEUTSCH

> "The public . . . demands certainties . . . , but there *are* no certainties."
> —H. L. Mencken (1880–1956)

Although the national public health system in the United States once dealt exclusively with the health problems of a small segment of the population (i.e., navy seamen), it is now responsible for the health of the entire U.S. population. This responsibility includes (*1*) attempting to prevent infectious diseases, chronic diseases, unintentional and violent injuries; (*2*) maintaining optimal occupational and environmental health; (*3*) addressing the health problems unique to minorities and special populations; (*4*) improving the population's access to health care; (*5*) providing some forms of health care; and (*6*) monitoring the quality of health care. These activities require considerable resources, and as the total expenditure on health care in the United States takes a larger share of the gross domestic product (currently about 14%), questions have been raised about the benefits derived from this investment (Gold et al., 1996). For example, there are large discrepancies in the success rates of surgical and other procedures from community to community, leading to questions as to whether the widespread use of many of these procedures is appropriate (Wennberg et al., 1989).

Questions about the return on investment (i.e., how "good" is a specific intervention, or health care in general) have forced public health officials to grapple with the problem of providing answers. Public health officials need to determine not only what constitutes appropriate care or a "worthwhile" intervention but also what is inappropriate. To accomplish this task, we need to decide what health outcomes society wants or needs, how we will measure these outcomes, and how we will place values on differences between outcomes. Although still important as a means of setting priorities and evaluating the effectiveness of interventions, mortality data are not a sufficiently complete measure of outcome; measures such as *quality-adjusted life-years* (QALYs) are rapidly becoming a standard measure of outcome. This chapter discusses some of the quantitative tools that are available to help public health decision makers understand the effectiveness and value of options available to them. It also describes some of the salient methodological questions that should be considered when using these tools.

Basic Questions and a List of Methods to Provide Answers

Tools used in decision analysis and economic evaluation have often evolved as pragmatic responses to answer specific questions. For example, an analyst could attempt to allocate health care resources in a manner that will maximize the value for society as a whole. Or, the problem and solution could focus on the minimization of medical care costs paid by a defined group. Diverse perspectives and lack of a single fundamental theoretical framework have created many methodological approaches. The roots of these approaches lie in diverse fields, such as operations research (engineering), valuation (economics and psychology), and distribution of goods (social welfare theory). In practice, valid methodological differences can yield different answers to what appear to be similar questions. For example, the results of cost-effectiveness analyses of mammography screening may vary from $8000 to $80,000 per life-year saved depending on perspective (e.g., society, payer, patient, or health care system), costs included (e.g., direct medical, direct nonmedical, productivity losses, and intangibles), type of cost data (e.g., charges and costs), discount rate used, and epidemiological characteristics (e.g., sensitivity and specificity of mammography, compliance, follow-up, and the population to be screened). Thus, both analysts and decision makers must be aware of the consequences of methodological choices. A series of basic questions must be answered at the start of an analysis of the effectiveness of a health intervention (Table 6.1). The following sections review methodological concerns in answering each question.

Magnitude of the Problem

The first step in evaluating interventions and setting priorities is to assess the magnitude of the impact of the health problem under consideration. This assessment can be done using the basic measures of mortality, morbidity, and cost (see Chapters 3 and 4). For mortality, commonly used measures include crude mortality rates, age-specific rates, and age-adjusted rates. Any of these measures can be applied to specific diseases or specific subpopulations and defined by certain

Table 6.1 Questions Decision Makers Need Answered and Methodological Approaches to Answering Them

Question to be Answered	Methods for Answering the Question
What is the magnitude of the health problem?	Descriptive epidemiology
How much of the problem is preventable?	Analytic epidemiology, (cohort studies)
How much of the problem can an intervention prevent?	Applied epidemiology (efficacy studies)
How much of the problem does an intervention prevent?	Applied epidemiology (effectiveness studies)
What does the intervention cost?	Cost analysis
What are the benefits and harms worth?	Outcome valuation
How should the costs, benefits, and hazards be combined?	Decision analysis and economic evaluation
What do additional resources buy?	Incremental analysis

variables (e.g., race, age, sex, income, education, and geographic location). Crude rates provide the best estimate of aggregate burden within a defined population, whereas age-adjusted rates are more suitable for making comparisons of mortality between different populations (Cates and Williamson, 1994).

Morbidity can be assessed by frequency (i.e., the incidence or prevalence), severity (e.g., case fatality rates), service utilization (e.g., physician visits or hospitalization), or disability (e.g., lost work time and functional status). To emphasize the importance of different conditions, the indicator that suggests the greatest disease or injury burden is often selected by advocates for specific interventions. Arthritis, for example, is a substantial health problem when assessed by disability (i.e., loss of function), but is a less significant condition when assessed by mortality. Single measures that combine mortality and morbidity have been developed to provide a more comprehensive picture of disease impact. Two examples of these measurements are QALYs and disability-adjusted life-years (DALYs). These measurements will be discussed later in this chapter.

Incidence and Prevalence Models

Prevalence describes what proportion of a defined population has a given disease or condition at one specific point in time or over a defined time period (i.e., a "snapshot"). Incidence describes the frequency of occurrence of new cases over a defined time period. Because some benefits of prevention programs accrue over extended periods of time, the use of incidence-based models to examine the impact of prevention programs is often more appropriate. For example, a hypertension control program enacted now may prevent stroke and ischemic heart disease events several years into the future.

Statistical Issue

Most burden of disease estimates are prevalence estimates. To calculate the costs and benefits of many interventions, however, an analyst often needs to know the incidence of disease (see Chapter 2). Assume, for example, that an intervention has been proposed that can prevent infection from a defined pathogen, but cannot cure those who are already infected (e.g., polio vaccination). Assessing the benefits of such an intervention will require measuring the incidence of the disease before and after the intervention. Incidence measures also are used in calculating the prevention and prevented fractions, discussed later in this chapter. Estimates of incidence and cumulative incidence from prevalence data can be calculated using the following standard equations, obtained from standard textbooks on epidemiology (e.g., Ahlbom and Norell, 1990; Rothman, 1986):

$$\text{Incidence} = P/\{(1 - P) \times D\} \qquad [6\text{--}1]$$

where P = prevalence,
$\quad D$ = average duration of the disease.

$$\text{Cumulative incidence} = 1 - e^{(-I \times t)} \qquad [6\text{--}2]$$

where t = total time period in which transmission/infection can occur
$\quad I$ = incidence,
$\quad e$ = the constant for natural logarithms ≈ 2.71828.

Attributable Risk

Attributable risk measures the amount of disease or injury that would be eliminated if a risk factor were eliminated from a defined population. Thus, it is a measure of the maximum benefit that an intervention can achieve. For example, the attributable risk of lung cancer associated with smoking cigarettes is equal to the reduction in lung cancer that would occur if nobody smoked in the defined population.

In the case of a single risk factor, the attributable risk (AR) associated with that factor is calculated as:

$$AR = \frac{(I_t - I_o)}{I_t} \qquad [6\text{--}3]$$

where I_t = the rate of occurrence (incidence as used here) among an exposed population, and I_o = the rate among the unexposed.

Alternatively, the AR can be calculated as:

$$AR = \frac{P_1(RR-1)}{1+P_1(RR-1)} \qquad [6\text{--}4]$$

where P_1 = the prevalence of the exposure, and RR = is the relative risk of the exposure.

For multiple exposures, or multiple strata of exposures, the AR can be expressed as:

$$AR = \frac{\sum\limits_{i=1}^{n}(P_i)(RR_i-1)}{1+\sum\limits_{i=1}^{n}(P_i)(RR_i-1)} \qquad [6\text{--}5]$$

where AR_j = the joint attributable risk, P_i = the proportion of population in each exposure stratum, RR_i = the relative risk associated with the exposures in each stratum, and n = number of strata.

In the case of multiple risk factors, one cannot calculate the total AR by simply summing the individual attributable risks for each risk factor calculated using Equation [6–3]. Since usually the risk factors are not independent. When there are multiple risk factors, Equation [6–4] provides a more accurate estimate of the AR. Equation [6–4], however, requires information on the frequency of exposure of persons in each stratum and the RR associated with each stratum.

Prevention and Prevented Fraction

Most interventions, including antismoking campaigns, do not achieve potential maximum benefits. Therefore, when evaluating prevention programs, the actual reduction in the incidence of disease resulting from the intervention is of interest. This can be determined from the *prevented fraction* (PF) as follows.

$$PF = \frac{I_o - I_T}{I_o} \qquad [6\text{--}6]$$

where I_o = the rate in the population without the intervention, and I_T = the rate in the population with the intervention.

Equation [6–6] can also be expressed as:

$$PF = P_1(1-RR) \qquad [6\text{--}7]$$

Efficacy and Effectiveness

Rarely does an intervention totally eliminate a risk factor. For example, whereas hypertension doubles the risk for mortality caused by coronary artery disease (CAD), clinical interventions to reduce blood pressure do not totally eliminate hypertension-related CAD mortality. Randomized controlled trials (RCTs) often provide the best estimates of what an intervention can achieve. This maximum possible reduction in incidence of a disease is termed the *efficacy* of an intervention (Haddix et al., 1996). This maximum impact (efficacy) is achieved when well-designed clinical trials include and involve carefully selected patients who will comply with the protocol and often lack related comorbidity. In most RCTs, participating clinicians are carefully selected for their interest in the problem and expertise, and they work with carefully trained staff who have time for follow-up and record keeping. These teams of clinicians and staff frequently have access to state-of-the-art equipment and work in top-of-the-line facilities.

In contrast to the idealized settings of most RCTs, in more routine clinical use, time is often constrained and all patients must be treated regardless of their willingness to comply with prescribed treatment regimens, or evidence of concurrent medical conditions. Therefore, in most cases the benefit obtained from an intervention applied in routine clinical or public health settings is less than the promise suggested by the controlled trials. The benefit that results from an intervention routinely applied to a population larger than that used in the RCTs is called *effectiveness.* The difference between efficacy and effectiveness can be significant, and obtaining realistic measures of effectiveness is difficult. Mandelblatt et al. (Gold et al., 1996) provide a more detailed discussion of obtaining estimates of effectiveness. They note that correcting for the tendency for RCTs to overestimate effectiveness is "problematic." A researcher may conduct an observational study after an intervention is introduced to determine the actual rate of effectiveness. In a preintervention situation, an analyst likely will have to resort to modeling to estimate the level of effectiveness, and conduct a number of sensitivity analyses (see later in this chapter) to determine the economic impact of various levels of effectiveness.

Recognizing Benefits and Harms in Effectiveness

Although the benefits of an intervention are often the focus when considering the term "effectiveness," the associated harms must also be recognized. However, many costs and harms may be hidden or less apparent, and thus not included in a cursory evaluation of an intervention. For example, in a mammography program, costs that may be overlooked or hard to measure include the time spent by the patients seeking mammography. Harms associated with mammography that are often, and incorrectly, ignored include the discomfort of the procedure, anxiety about the results (which are often false-positive), discomfort from any follow-up biopsies, and anxiety while waiting for results from the biopsies. Many public health interventions are population-based programs, in which the harms and costs are accrued by large groups of subjects, most of whom do not have or will not get the disease or condition that is the target of the program. The benefits, however, may only affect a few persons who will avoid contracting the disease or condition as a result of the program. Therefore, it is important to fully assess *(1)* the magnitude and severity of both the benefits and the harms and *(2)* who accrues these benefits and harms. The overall "balance" (i.e., do the benefits outweigh the harms for society?) must then be compared (Coughlin and Beauchamp, 1996).

Decision Analysis

Decision analysis is a framework that public health officials can use to measure the benefits and harms of one or more interventions. Decision analyses have tremendous power to help sort through options, identify critical gaps in information (i.e., research needs), and be adapted to meet the needs of specific communities or populations. They facilitate decisions even in the face of uncertainty. One of the most common methodologies used in decision analysis is the decision tree (Haddix et al., 1996). A brief outline of some of the steps involved in building a decision tree and some of the quantitative problems that can arise follows. The points itemized in the outline are illustrated in a case study of a decision analysis of the prevention of Lyme disease after tick bites (Magid et al., 1992).

Outline for Building a Decision Tree

- List all appropriate options for intervention. Two or more interventions can be evaluated in a side-by-side comparison. It is *always* appropriate to consider including the "do-nothing" option. The do-nothing option must be included if only one intervention is being evaluated.
- Decide on the *unit of outcome.* The appropriate unit is dependent on the perspective of the target audience. For example, clinicians primarily may be interested in clinical and epidemiological parameters (e.g., cases averted and reduction in mortality), whereas policy makers and analysts may emphasize the need to have the benefits and harms measured in economic terms (e.g., dollars). The "construction rules" below contain an important rule related to outcomes.
- Construct a *decision tree.* A decision tree is a skeleton, or schematic diagram, that presents all the options being studied and all the different paths that pa-

tients or populations may follow to end-up at one of the outcomes that may occur if an intervention were used. The first set of *"branches"* in the tree are the interventions being studied (Fig. 6.1). Thereafter, the branches from each option are dependent on intervention-specific factors (e.g., characteristics of the population, results of diagnostic tests, number of potential outcomes from applying the intervention, and risk of adverse events). Each time a branch splits into two or more possible occurrences, the point of splitting is termed a *"probability node."* For the strategy labeled "test," the first proba-bility node depends on the probability of a patient with a tick bite presenting with a rash (erythema migrans) indicative of Lyme disease (Fig. 6.1). Those persons without a rash are serologically tested, and the tree branch divides into two branches labeled "test positive" or "test negative." The final out-comes are placed at the end of each final branch, and are termed the *terminal nodes.* In Figure 6.1, the final outcomes are clinical outcomes and do *not* in-dicate any valuation of each outcome.

- Attach probabilities to each branch. In general, every time a node occurs, a probability must be attached to each branch that splits off from that node. The probability associated with the branch labeled "no rash" in Figure 6.1 is 0.979, and the probabilities of "test positive" and "test negative" are each 0.50. The probabilities associated with each branch can be obtained from many sources (e.g., published studies, meta-analyses, program evaluation information, and expert opinion). (See also the "construction rules" below for a decision-tree rule related to probabilities).

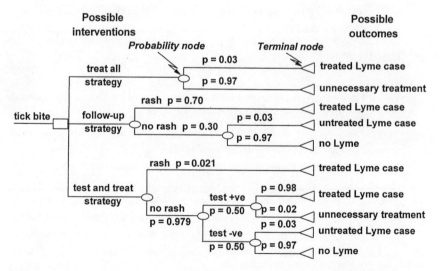

Figure 6.1. An example of a decision tree: determining the optimal treatment for Lyme disease after a tick bite. Note: for simplicity, the probabilities for the "test and treat" strat-egy do not include the probabilities of patients returning for treatment, which were in-cluded in the original study. [Adapted from Magid et al., 1992.]

- Calculate the *expected values* for each option. This is done by multiplying and adding, or *"folding back,"* the values of the outcomes by the probabilities along the branches. This procedure provides a single estimate of the expected value associated with each option. For example, in Figure 6.1, the expected probability of successfully identifying *and* treating a case of Lyme disease under the "test and treat" strategy is: probability of treating a case or a case patient with Lyme disease with "no rash" plus probability of treating a case or case patient of Lyme disease with "rash":

$$(0.98 \times 0.50 \times 0.979) + (0.021) = 0.50071$$

The outcome of this option can be compared with those from the other two strategies in Case Study 6.1

- Two "construction rules" for decision trees. First, the probabilities for all the branches that split from a given node must sum to 1. Second, the outcomes must be both exhaustive and mutually exclusive. That is, all possible options must be listed, and each individual that may face the options can only reach one outcome.

Case Study 6.1: Prevention of Lyme Disease after Tick Bites: A Case Study Using Decision Trees

Magid et al. (1992) used a simple decision tree (Fig. 6.1) to determine which of three strategies was the optimal treatment for a hypothetical cohort of 100,000 persons bitten by *Ixodes* ticks in an area where Lyme disease is "common." The three strategies were: (*1*) treat all, which treats patients with tick bites for 2 weeks with antibiotics; (*2*) test and treat, which treats only those patients who have a rash (erythema migrans) symptomatic of Lyme disease, or those who test positive after a serological test; and (*3*) follow-up, which treats only those patients who have a rash. To make the outcomes both exhaustive and complete (one of the "construction rules" for decision trees), the possible outcomes have been simplified. For example, in Figure 6.1 note that there is no possibility of unsuccessfully treating Lyme disease. This is an example of decision analysts balancing reality with usability, and acknowledging the limitations of available data.

Probabilities were obtained from published studies and expert opinion. In addition to the "best estimate" of a given probability, "plausible ranges" are provided, which are used for sensitivity analyses. The outcomes listed in Figure 6.1 are clinical, and all that can be done is to consider the probability of each outcome occurring under each strategy. To compare strategies, the outcomes must be converted into a common unit, or metric. Magid et al. did this by placing a cost on each of the outcomes, and then comparing the average cost per patient accrued under each strategy. They collected data for the costs from a variety of sources. The amount of medical services used by patients diagnosed with Lyme disease was determined by sampling medical charts of patients. Also, experts in the field of Lyme disease were interviewed concerning the amount of services required. Estimates of the charges for laboratory tests, physician services, hospital costs, and hospital medications

were obtained from an insurance company. Ten pharmacies were surveyed to obtain estimates of the charges associated with antibiotics. The assessment of the costs of untreated
Lyme disease were limited to those costs associated with short and intermediate sequelae
(i.e., <1 year). Thus, the costs over time were not discounted (see text for an explanation of
discounting).

Using the baseline assumptions, the "treat-all" strategy provides the lowest average
charge per patient; with the "follow-up" strategy the second least expensive. Sensitivity
analyses found that, at a 0.03 (3%) probability of infection from a tick bite, the conclusions
did not change over the full range of reasonable values for costs.

One of the limitations of the study is that it used charges, which usually contain profits,
rather than actual costs. Furthermore, other economic costs (e.g., travel costs incurred by
patients and the value of lost productivity) were not included. Thus, in reality, the perspective of the study is from that of the payer. The authors of the study readily acknowledge
these limitations in their discussion of their results, and claimed that using actual costs, and
incorporating other economic costs, would not likely change the overall conclusion.

The Importance of Sensitivity Analyses

Decision trees requires use of quantitative data, yet estimates of probabilities and
the values of outcomes often are uncertain. Thus, sensitivity analyses must be
conducted to evaluate how *robust* the initial results are. Sensitivity analyses can
be *univariate* (i.e., changing one variable) or *multivariate* (i.e., two or more variables altered simultaneously). Within those two broad categories, there are many
types of sensitivity analyses. An analysis can be "worst case" or "best case," or it
can consist of altering predefined parameters by given amounts or percentages.
The amount by which a given parameter is altered may be based on some known
data or on some arbitrary amount set by the analyst. More sophisticated methodologies for sensitivity analyses include Monte Carlo simulations, in which the
amount by which a parameter is increased or decreased is dependent on some previously defined probability distribution. Several hundred iterations are run to provide a probability distribution of expected values.

However, these forms of sensitivity analyses depend on both a combination of
data and the judgment of the analyst as to how much a value might differ. *Threshold analysis* is a form of sensitivity analysis that removes the subjective element
of the analyst's judgment. The goal of threshold analysis is to find the value of a
key parameter that will cause the conclusion to change, which is equivalent to the
"testing to destruction or change" concept used in engineering.

To illustrate threshold analysis, consider the following hypothetical example:
for a given infectious disease, an analyst may compare a proposed large-scale,
screen-and-treat program to a treat-all program, with the measure of outcome being the cost per actual case successfully treated (note that the do-nothing option is
not valid because one program definitely will be implemented). Based on some

expert opinion, the analyst assumed that the test will have a sensitivity (i.e., probability of giving a true-positive result) of 95%. The initial results of the decision-tree analysis determined that the screen-and-treat option provides the highest expected value (i.e., had the lowest cost per case successfully treated). Threshold analysis, however, determines that the screen-and-treat option only provides the lowest cost per case successfully treated if the sensitivity of the screening test is 90% or greater. That is, with a sensitivity of 90% or less, the treat-all option would be preferred. The question then becomes: how realistic is it to expect the test to be 90% sensitive "in the field"? This is an example of how results from threshold analyses can help define critical gaps in a database, and thus help prioritize applied research agendas.

Other Forms of Decision Analysis

Decision trees are not the only methodology for conducting decision analysis. For example, screening for cervical cancer may be done annually or less frequently, but the probability of a positive or a negative result is dependent on the results of previous tests. The process may be best analyzed using *Markov models*. Mandelblatt et al. (Gold et al., 1996) discuss Markov and other types of models that may be used in a cost-effectiveness analysis. Modeling is as much of an art as a science, and often, more than one method can be used to model a particular problem. The choice of model depends on many factors, with one of the most important being the ability of the intended audience to both understand and accept the results.

Economic Evaluation: Conducting a Prevention Effectiveness Study

In choosing between options, or to evaluate a single intervention, decision trees are often used as part of a quantitative economic analysis. Economic evaluations focus on "true" or *opportunity* costs. An opportunity cost is the valuation of an input in terms of the alternative uses for that input. Also valued are those resources that may not incur a direct payment (e.g., time off work). Furthermore, an effort is made to place a dollar value on intangible factors (e.g., pain and fear).

Financial Versus Economic Analyses

The differences between economic analyses and financial analyses commonly cause confusion. A financial analysis is an accounting approach, wherein the analysis is restricted to actual cash charges and direct, cash-valued benefits. An economic analysis uses the "true," or opportunity, costs. The choice between economic or financial analyses determines the type of data required. For example, suppose an economic analysis is being conducted on an intervention that requires a patient to make repeated visits to a medical facility. The amount of time each visit takes should be measured or estimated and valued. Such data would not be required in a purely financial analysis of the intervention.

The actual type of analysis chosen will largely depend on the target audience and the perspective. Because economic analyses more fully reflect the complete costs and benefits to society, decision analyses of public health programs should be conducted using an economic analytic framework. More information is provided later in this chapter concerning how to collect economic costs rather than financial charges. Concurrent with the decision on the type of analysis, an analyst should choose the *method* of analysis.

Three Methods for Economic Evaluation

Three methods primarily are used in prevention effectiveness: *cost-benefit analysis (CBA)*, *cost-effectiveness analysis (CEA)*, and *cost-utility analysis (CUA)* (Table 6.2). Some texts include cost analysis as a fourth method. However, cost analysis is a limited approach to resource allocations because it does not include estimates of the benefits associated with an intervention. Furthermore, obtaining all costs is an essential part of the three methods listed here. Because of these shortcomings, cost analysis is not included as a distinct method suitable for setting health care priorities.

Cost-Benefit Analysis
For many applied economists, this method is considered the "gold standard" by which all other methods are judged. In its simplest form, a cost-benefit analysis

Table 6.2 Three Methods of Conducting an Economic Analysis

Method of Analysis	Included Costs*		Outcome Measure* (Benefit)	Summary Measure
	Direct	*Indirect*		
Cost-Benefit	Yes	Yes	Dollars	Net present value
Cost-Effectiveness	Yes	Often	Health outcome[†]	Cost-effectiveness ratio
Cost-Utility	Yes	Occasionally	Utility measure[‡]	Cost-utility ratio

*All future costs and benefits, monetary and nonmonetary, should be discounted to year zero.

[†]An example of a health outcome is cases averted.

[‡]An example of a utility measure is a quality-adjusted-life year (QALY).

lists all the costs and benefits that might occur as a result of an intervention over the prespecified, analytic time horizon. These costs and benefits are discounted to the *year zero* (Haddix et al., 1996). If the total discounted benefits are greater than the total discounted costs, then the intervention is said to have a positive *net present value (NPV),* which is calculated as follows:

$$NPV = \sum_{t=0}^{t=n} \frac{(\text{benefits} - \text{costs})_t}{(1+r)^t} \qquad [6\text{--}8]$$

where t = year, from 0, . . . , n; n = number of years being evaluated; r = discount rate.

CBA is most useful under three circumstances. The first is when a choice has to be made between two or more options. In such a case, the logical action is to give top priority to those options that give the highest positive NPVs. Second, the results of a CBA analysis also can indicate the economic impact of a single intervention. Third, CBA is useful because it can include an array of substantial benefits or costs not directly associated with a health outcome (e.g., time off from work taken by family members to care for sick relatives). One of the most important quantitative issues associated with CBA is that all costs and benefits must be expressed in monetary terms, including the value of human lives lost or saved as a result of the intervention. Quantifying all benefits and costs is not a trivial task (see section Approaches to Estimating the Value of Health and Nonhealth Outcomes, later in this chapter).

Cost-Effectiveness Analysis

A cost-effectiveness analysis expresses the net direct and indirect costs and cost savings in terms of a predefined unit of health outcome (e.g., lives saved and cases of illness avoided). It is probably the most frequently used method in prevention effectiveness. The method can be expressed as:

Total net cost = Cost of intervention + Cost of side effects of intervention − Cost of disease averted − Indirect costs

When divided by the number of health outcomes averted (i.e., the denominator), the result becomes the total net cost per unit health outcome (e.g., total net cost per death averted). Many of the data required for an economic CEA, with a societal perspective, are the same as for a CBA, with the most important exception being the avoidance of valuing a human life. Explicitly or implicitly, the value of a human life is part of the health outcome used (e.g., lives saved). An explanation of the type of costs that are included is provided later, as is a discussion on *cost-effectiveness ratios.*

A distinct limitation of CEA is that there is no numerical valuation of the actual health outcome. For example, CEA can only provide estimates of the net costs of averting a case of polio or averting a migraine headache. CEA cannot provide any information as to how society might value each averted case, even in a seemingly similar outcome (e.g., influenza in a person 75 years versus influenza in an infant). Thus, CEA is best used when comparing two or more strategies or interventions that have the same health outcome. For example, is vaccination more cost effective than chemoprophylaxis in preventing a case of influenza? CEA can also be used to explicitly define the cost of a single intervention per single health outcome. Such an answer may be useful when making policy decisions concerning the implementation of an intervention.

Cost-Utility Analysis

CUA is a specialized form of CEA, where the outcome is measured, or valued, in terms of utility for the quality of life resulting from a given health outcome. Unlike CEA, CUA attempts to differentiate between the quality associated with an averted case of polio and an averted migraine headache. Examples of units of valuation include the QALY (Patrick and Erickson, 1993) and disability-adjusted life years (DALY) (Murray, 1994).

Similar to CEA, in CUA the value of life itself is implicit in the denominator (e.g., calculation of a QALY requires the valuation of life). One unresolved quantitative issue, however, is how to deal with time costs (e.g., time lost from work as a result of illness). Some authors state explicitly that productivity losses should not be included in the numerator unless "the utility measurement in the denominator [e.g., QALYs] does not incorporate productivity losses," (Dasbach and Teutsch, 1996). Other authors (Garber et al., 1996) state that no convention exists regarding the placement of such morbidity costs, but they also note that such costs should not be accounted for twice. Thus, when conducting a CUA, the analyst should explicitly state if morbidity costs (e.g., lost productivity) are included in the numerator.

QALYs: A Brief Explanation

Quality-adjusted life years are a combination of the utility of a given health state and the length of life lived under that health state. The utility of a health state is commonly measured on a continuous scale from zero to one, where zero represents death and one represents perfect health. Values of the utility of a defined health state can be obtained by using one of three methodologies: expert opinion, values from previous studies, and surveys. The latter method can be divided into two categories, *direct* and *indirect*. A brief discussion of survey techniques from both categories follows; a more comprehensive review can be found in Patrick and Erickson (1993).

Direct Surveys of Utilities

Techniques for directly soliciting utility evaluations via surveys include the *standard gamble*, *time trade-off*, and the use of a *rating scale*. The standard gamble provides a probability-weighted average utility (i.e., the expected utility) for a set of health outcomes. In practice, an individual is asked to choose between two options. One option is a gamble, and represents, for example, a medical intervention with a probability (p) of death and a probability ($1-p$) of healthy life. The other option, which has perfect certainty, is to live a defined number of years with a chronic condition, in less than perfect health. The probabilities are systematically changed until the person is indifferent between the two options. At the point of indifference, the expected value of the gamble option is assumed to be equal to the utility of the health state in the other option.

In a time–trade-off exercise, a person is asked to choose between living in a chronic state of health for a defined number of years or living in perfect health (and then dying) for a shorter period. The difference in time lived in each state is altered until the individual is indifferent. Note that the time–trade-off exercise does not ask the respondent to evaluate probabilities, as each outcome is presented as a certainty. The final method of directly surveying utilities is to use a rating scale, on which an individual directly marks on a scale of, for example, 0–100 how they value a specified health outcome.

These methods can be problematic. First, each method is a simplification of the number of options/outcomes facing the patient. Furthermore, the methodologies deliberately limit the respondents' ability to state how they may value the limited set of outcomes offered for consideration. The standard gamble also assumes that respondents can readily evaluate the probabilities assigned to the gamble. The time–trade-off methodology implicitly assumes that respondents will not undervalue, or even ignore, years of life lived at the end of a life span. Thus, the three methods essentially ask respondents three different types of questions. Exemplifying this difference, the correlation between the standard gamble and time–trade-off has ranged from 0.31–0.65 (Gold et al., 1996). Another problem is that interviewers can influence the answers given. Furthermore, the same respondent tested twice may not give the same response both times. Overall, these problems can result in different values being obtained by using different methods, or in values that may not be readily replicated between studies even if the same method is used.

To expand the ability of a respondent to state how they value a given outcome, *multiattribute questionnaires* (i.e., the indirect approach) have been developed. These divide a health state into subgroups, or *domains,* that can be later added together to give a single health-utility number. Examples of these domains include opportunity (e.g., social and cultural), health perceptions (i.e., self-satisfaction with health state), functional status (i.e., limitations to usual work and social roles), psychological function (e.g., depression and alertness), and physical function (e.g., mobility and self-care). Within each domain, a respondent must rate the impact of the disease from a set of descriptions. For example, in the domain of mobility, respondents might state that they are able to walk around their house and neighborhood without help, but with some limitations. This response is assigned a preference weight (e.g., 0.9) on a scale of 0–1. The preference-weighted responses from all the other domains are then used to construct a single utility index by using a predetermined equation. The key to such a system, however, is determining the appropriate set of preference weights for each response within each domain. Unless weights from other studies or investigator preferences are used, the key to setting such weights is to identify an appropriate group of "judges," and use methods such as the time–trade-off to elicit weights from this group. With this method, health state preferences have been shown to be "remarkably stable" across different populations (Patrick and Erickson, 1993).

The use of health utilities is not without problems. One key problem is that both the direct and indirect techniques focus on long-term disabilities. QALYs, therefore, may not be an appropriate tool to measure the impact of diseases that cause short-duration morbidity among substantial numbers of a population (e.g., influenza and dengue fever). Another problem is that different studies may use different methods to evaluate the utility of a given health state, and results may differ quite markedly, causing notably different conclusions regarding the cost utility of an intervention. For example, Gill and Feinstein (1994) evaluated 75 published articles that used one or more quality-of-life instruments, and identified a total of 159 different instruments used in these studies. A related problem is that of comparison between noticeably different diseases and health states. For example, the loss of utility due to diabetes may not be comparable to the loss of utility due to angina. The perspective of the user of QALYs is also important. Results from a clinical trial that measures outcomes of an intervention in QALYs may only be applicable to the small set of patients included in the trial. For a policymaker, QALYs derived from a clinical trial may not provide sufficient information regarding the potential returns when an intervention is used in a large population (O'Brien et al., 1997). In summary, one QALY is not automatically equal to another QALY. The danger is that "league tables," which attempt to rank interventions by cost-utility results, may be constructed without regard to the differences that result from estimation techniques and natural differences in disease states.

Choosing an Analytic Method

Choosing an analytic method will be influenced by the following five points. Each point should be fully addressed before the start of an economic evaluation.

1. *Define the question and the intended audience for the answer.* As noted earlier, this step helps define and refine both the type of study (e.g., financial, economic, and socioeconomic) and the methodology (e.g., CBA, CEA, or CUA). Many studies attempt to answer too many questions at once, which confuses readers. *Stakeholders* are usually the readers most interested in the answer. A stakeholder is defined as a person or group that may have a vested interest in seeing the intervention deployed (or even preventing the intervention from being deployed). Examples of stakeholders for public health interventions include government public health officials, politicians, persons suffering from the disease or condition that the intervention aims to alleviate, private firms producing the intervention (e.g., pharmaceutical companies), nongovernment aid agencies, providers, health insurance firms, and advocacy groups.

2. *Decide on the perspective.* The perspective defines those costs and benefits that are included in a study. Only those costs and benefits directly accrued by members of the chosen perspective are included in the study. To help decide the appropriate perspective, determine who will pay for the costs and consequences of the intervention. The list of potential perspectives include the patient, the payer, the provider, the health care system, and society. Some perspectives include other perspectives as a subset. For example, the societal perspective usually includes all other perspectives as subsets, whereas the health care system perspective may include only the payer and the provider. The choice of perspective will often depend on the question and the intended audience. Whenever interventions will use societal resources (e.g., tax revenues), the societal perspective should be used.

3. *List other possible interventions.* Although the potential audience may focus on the economics of a particular intervention, including other practical interventions in a study will allow an analysis of the incremental costs and benefits associated with the interventions. The do-nothing option should also be considered for inclusion, because it can be used to illustrate both the burden imposed by the disease and the magnitude of the benefits from deploying an intervention.

4. *Decide on the health outcome of interest.* Potential health outcomes include cases averted, lives saved, years of healthy life saved, treatments prevented, QALYs gained, and DALYs gained. The choice will partly depend on the question, audience, perspective, and analytic method. For example, a hospital administrator may be most interested in treatments prevented, because this would represent potential financial losses. Conversely, a health insurance company may consider reduced number of treatments a savings. When a societal perspective is the focus of the study, the Panel on Cost-Effectiveness in Health and Medicine, convened by the U.S. Public Health Service in 1993, recently recommended that prevention effectiveness studies use QALYs almost exclusively as the health outcome (Gold et al., 1996). This recommendation

stems from a desire to have a ready comparison between interventions for vastly different diseases and conditions. However, as acknowledged by some panel members, the concept of QALYs is not without controversy.

5. *Determine the time frame and discount rate.* Although the choice of the time frame for the intervention is often obvious, the choice of the analytic time frame is dependent on the analyst's interpretation of how long the costs and benefits will "linger." For example, in a vaccination campaign of a cohort of children, the direct medical costs may be distributed over a relatively short period (e.g., 2 years). Some other costs may be generated over time, such as the costs of care associated with those children that develop long-term sequelae in reaction to either the vaccine or the disease itself. The benefits, however, may accrue over many years in the form of reduced mortality and morbidity. Thus, the time frame should be sufficiently long to capture all the significant costs and benefits.

All costs and benefits that accrue after 1 year should be discounted back to the base year. Discounting reflects the fact that individuals and societies would prefer to, or must, consume goods and services now rather than delay consumption to a future date. For example, most persons would prefer to be paid a dollar now rather than to wait for 1 year. Discounting is not done to merely allow for inflation. Even if there were 0% inflation, future benefits and costs must still be discounted so as to allow for the preference for benefits now rather than in the future. Health outcomes must also be discounted. That is, a healthy-life-year saved now is usually worth more now than a healthy-life-year saved 10 years from now. The formula for discounting costs and benefits is given in Equation 6–8, above.

A crucial consideration when discounting is choosing the appropriate discount rate. The higher the rate, the smaller the present value of future costs and benefits. The Panel on Cost-Effectiveness in Health and Medicine recommended that a discount rate of 3% be used when conducting a prevention effectiveness study with a societal perspective (Lipscomb et al., 1996). It further recommended that sensitivity analyses be conducted using other discount rates (e.g., 0%, 5%, and 8%). If the perspective of a study is not societal, then selecting a different discount rate may be appropriate. For example, when conducting a study from the perspective of private businesses, using a rate equal to the "prime rate" charged by banks to certain customers may be an appropriate discount rate.

Approaches to Estimating the Value of Health and Nonhealth Outcomes

In a prevention effectiveness setting, the economic impact of a disease or condition can be assessed using two methods. These are the *cost-of-illness* (COI) method and the *willingness-to-pay* (WTP) approach. The COI methodology collects and uses data concerning direct medical costs, direct nonmedical costs and productivity losses, or indirect nonmedical costs. An appendix listing sources for collecting COI data has been published (Haddix et al., 1996). These sources include literature reviews, national databases, publications such as *Health United States* (published by the U.S. Department of Health and Human Services), and databases from the private sector (e.g., The Medstat Group).

The WTP approach estimates what an individual or society would be willing to pay to avoid contracting a given disease or condition. The WTP approach goes beyond the COI methodology in that it implicitly values the *intangible costs and benefits* of an intervention (e.g., fear and pain). Furthermore, a WTP approach can value nonhealth benefits that might arise from a health intervention, such as the value of clean air (no smog) resulting from a program to reduce air pollution. Such valuations are often obtained directly through surveys, although indirect methods are available. A typical WTP survey obtains sociodemographic information (e.g., education, income, age, and sex) and data regarding respondents' knowledge of and attitude towards the problem. Respondents are given a hypothetical scenario regarding an intervention (e.g., "Suppose a vaccine was available to protect against disease X"). Respondents are then asked what is the maximum that they would be willing to pay for the intervention. This maximum amount could be solicited either as a single, open-ended question (e.g., "What is the maximum that you would be willing to pay?"), or respondents could be given a set amount and asked if they would pay that amount (e.g., "Would you be willing to pay Y dollars?"). The latter technique can be made more sophisticated by randomly assigning each respondent to one of several different set amounts. An analysis of the distribution of percentage of positive responses versus the amount "offered" can provide a decision maker with a picture of how persons value an intervention over a wide range of values. By using statistical models, analysts can obtain an understanding of how valuations are influenced by sociodemographics, knowledge, and attitudes.

Categorizing Costs

Costs can be categorized as *direct medical, direct nonmedical,* and *indirect costs of lost productivity.* Direct medical costs include those medical costs for delivering an intervention (e.g., drugs and physician time) and the costs of medical care (e.g., medical buildings, medical machinery, maintenance) saved by averting a case of disease. Direct nonmedical costs are those costs associated with the treatment (e.g., transportation and child-care costs). Productivity losses include items such as patient time spent traveling to a clinic for treatment and time away from work.

Costs also can be categorized as either *variable* or *fixed.* Variable costs are those costs that vary depending on the numbers of persons treated or units of interventions delivered (e.g., cost of drugs administered). Fixed costs are those costs that do

not vary in the short to medium term (e.g., cost of a building). One set of cost terminology, appropriate for the audience, should be used throughout a single study.

An additional category of costs, labeled *intangible* costs, includes those items
for which a widely accepted value is often difficult to find. Examples of such
items are pain, fear, and suffering. The WTP approach of costing health outcomes
can be used to obtain values for such items. However, if a cost-of-illness approach is used, then researchers may resort to simply listing the number of readily identifiable intangible costs and benefits that may be associated with an intervention. These non–dollar valued costs and benefits may become crucial in the
public debate concerning the adoption of a particular intervention. Thus, the researcher should acknowledge the existence of such intangibles without being ob-
ligated to attach an unsubstantiated dollar value. Haddix et al. (1996) provide an
expanded definition of all of these costs and give a detailed list of examples of
costs (see Haddix et al., 1996; Table 8.1).

Sources for Obtaining Economic Costs

Decision analyses of public health programs should use economic costs (i.e., opportunity costs). However, financial charge data (e.g., the price of drugs bought at
a for-profit pharmacy) are often more readily available. The analyst can obtain estimates of the economic costs in several ways. Large-volume discount prices can
be used as proxies for opportunity costs. For example, the U.S. federal government sets the amount of money that it will reimburse for Medicare-related hospital inpatient care, reported by diagnosis-related groups (DRGs). These amounts,
and amendments to the list of DRGs, are usually published annually in the *Federal Register* by the Health Care Financing Administration (HCFA) of the Department of Health and Human Services [e.g., *Federal Register,* Vol. 61 (170):
46166–46328, 1996]. The same source also provides a list of average cost-to-
charge ratios for urban and rural hospitals (Table 6.3). These ratios allow a researcher to take hospital charges, such as those published annually in *Health
United States* (National Center for Health Statistics, 1997) and convert them into
estimates of economic costs. Haddix et al. (1996) provide a detailed list of other
sources for collecting cost-of-illness data.

However, such databases have limitations. Many databases report average cost
per procedure but not the cost per case of disease. For example, a researcher may
readily find the Medicaid national average reimbursement for an office visit, or an
x-ray, but may have difficulty finding data concerning the "average" cost of a case
of a disease (e.g., what is the average cost for a patient who is diagnosed with
Lyme disease, and who is cured with a 2 week course of antibiotics?). The researcher can model such a cost by making some assumptions regarding the number of physician visits required, the number and type of diagnostic tests that may

Table 6.3. Statewide Average Operating Cost-to-Charge Ratios for Urban and Rural Hospitals (Case Weighted), August 1996*

State	Urban	Rural
Alabama	0.0420	0.476
Alaska	0.505	0.796
Arizona	0.423	0.568
Arkansas	0.540	0.495
California	0.405	0.540
Colorado	0.513	0.604
Connecticut	0.553	0.551
Delaware	0.503	0.500
District of Columbia	0.525	—
Florida	0.414	0.418
Georgia	0.527	0.532
Hawaii	0.484	0.567
Idaho	0.580	0.635
Illinois	0.478	0.599
Indiana	0.564	0.613
Iowa	0.540	0.684
Kansas	0.449	0.649
Kentucky	0.506	0.574
Louisiana	0.475	0.540
Maine	0.593	0.570
Maryland	0.765	0.816
Massachusetts	0.574	0.600
Michigan	0.489	0.594
Minnesota	0.563	0.641
Mississippi	0.525	0.527
Missouri	0.459	0.529
Montana	0.513	0.615
Nebraska	0.526	0.684
Nevada	0.321	0.563
New Hampshire	0.591	0.611
New Jersey	0.479	—
New Mexico	0.484	0.546
New York	0.584	0.679
North Carolina	0.539	0.498
North Dakota	0.651	0.694
Ohio	0.557	0.594
Oklahoma	0.489	0.558
Oregon	0.577	0.671
Pennsylvania	0.436	0.580
Puerto Rico	0.495	0.643
Rhode Island	0.587	—
South Carolina	0.477	0.501
South Dakota	0.559	0.648
Tennessee	0.536	0.572
Texas	0.462	0.565
Utah	0.462	0.675
Vermont	0.576	0.587
Virginia	0.499	0.536
Washington	0.634	0.688
West Virginia	0.578	0.542
Wisconsin	0.604	0.665
Wyoming	0.495	0.734

*From *Federal Register*, 1996.

be ordered, and the type of antibiotics prescribed. Each of these components can then be priced using average costs, or Medicare-allowable rates. Such a model is not certain to reflect actual average costs. The researcher, however, knowing the elements used to construct such an estimate, can conduct sensitivity analyses to determine the impact of increases or decreases in the cost of an illness .

Another limitation of many of the cost databases is that they only report average costs. The distribution of cost data is *not* likely to be normally distributed (i.e., do not have a "bell-shaped" distribution curve; see Chapter 2), and median costs are often much lower than average costs. Thus, average costs may overstate the costs accrued by a patient with a "typical" case of a given disease. Both of these data-related problems are particularly important to researchers who need to evaluate the economic impact of a disease. Such evaluations are crucial when examining the economics associated with an intervention designed to lower the incidence and prevalence of a disease. In such a situation, researchers often must conduct original research (e.g., examining medical charts and conducting interviews) to obtain relevant cost data. Databases and tapes can be bought from many sources (see Haddix et al., 1996) that do list the costs accrued by individual patients using the International Classification of Diseases-9 (ICD-9) codes.

None of these methods of obtaining costs are necessarily quick, easy, or inexpensive. One of the fundamental lessons of prevention effectiveness research is that the same level of planning and thought devoted to collecting epidemiological data must also be devoted to the collection of economic data.

Cost-Effectiveness Ratios

Once cost and benefit data have been obtained, cost-effectiveness ratios can be calculated for each of the three methodologies. For CBA, the present value of the benefits can be divided by the present value of the costs to give the *benefit-cost ratio (BCR)*. The problem with the BCR is that, although it provides an estimate of the return (i.e., benefit) obtained for each dollar of cost, it does not provide a sense of perspective. Thus, although a BCR of 6.5:1 indicates that there are $6.50 of benefits for each $1 of costs, there is no indication of how much the intervention actually costs. Thus, the present value of both the costs and benefits must be reported, as well as the resultant NPV.

Three different ratios can be used to calculate CEA: *average cost* per unit of health outcome, the *marginal cost* of an additional unit of health outcome, and the *incremental cost* per unit of health outcome. The average cost is the total cost of an intervention divided by the total number of health outcomes provided by the intervention. The marginal cost is the cost of obtaining one extra unit of health outcome. For example, if a planned intervention is estimated to save 150 lives, at an average cost of *X* dollars per life saved, what would be the cost of saving the 151st life?

Table 6.4 A Hypothetical Example of Incremental Cost-Effectiveness Analysis

Strategy*	Cases Occurring per 1000 Treated	Cost per 1000 Treated	Average Cost per Case Treated	Additional Cases Prevented (A)	Additional Costs (B)	Incremental CE Ratio: Cost per Case Prevented (B/A)
1	30.9	$2278	$73.72			
2	19.0	$5341	$281.11	11.9	$3063	$257.39
3	7.2	$7866	$1092.50	11.8	$2525	$213.98

*Additional cases prevented are calculated strategy 1 minus strategy 2 and strategy 2 minus strategy 3. Similar calculations were made for additional costs.

An example will illustrate the value of an incremental analysis (see Table 6.4). Based on the number of cases occurring, three strategies (i.e., interventions) are ranked from least effective (strategy 1) to most effective (strategy 3). However, the costs of the intervention programs in strategy 2 and 3 are such that strategy 1 is cheaper in terms of average cost per case treated. This average is misleading because a researcher cannot determine the cost of averting a case. By calculating the incremental cost of each case prevented (Table 6.4), it can be seen that the price of switching from strategy 1 to strategy 2 is $257.39 per additional case averted. Similarly, switching from strategy 2 to strategy 3 would cost an additional $213.98 per additional case averted, and going directly from strategy 1 to strategy 3 would cost $235.69 per additional case averted. The question is: "Would it be worthwhile to employ either strategy 2 or strategy 3 instead of strategy 1?" (See the sections Resource Allocation and Valuing Outcomes, below.)

The cost-effective ratios for CUA are similar to those used for CEA, with the exception that the outcome is always in a utility measure. For example, one can calculate average cost per QALY saved, or compare the incremental cost ratio between two or more interventions in terms of incremental dollars per QALY saved (see Case Study 6.2).

Case Study 6.2: The Economics of Different Strategies to Ensure Folic Acid Intake

Folic acid can reduce the risk for neural tube defects. Kelly et al. (1996) assessed alternative strategies for ensuring adequate intake (i.e., 0.4 mg/day) of folic acid for women of childbearing age. A decision tree was constructed to evaluate the following interventions:

1. Baseline—no program
2. Fortification from 0.07–0.70 mg/100 gm of cereal grains
3. Oral supplementation with folic acid tablets for women of childbearing age

A societal perspective was used and the results were expressed as the incremental cost effectiveness per life-year saved and incremental cost per QALY saved. The analysis assessed the benefits (i.e., reduced neural tube defects) and the harms (i.e., impairing the ability to diagnose vitamin B_{12} deficiency) for each strategy. The baseline levels of folic acid intake were calculated from the National Health and Nutrition Examination Survey consumption information. Incidence rates were derived from surveillance systems. Efficacy information was derived from randomized, controlled trials. Compliance with supplementation was based on expert opinion. The costs of illness were obtained from medical-claims data and previous studies that had determined excess school education and institutional costs associated with children who have neural tube defects. Implementation costs for each strategy were determined from Food and Drug Administration (FDA) estimates and health promotion experts. Health outcomes were assessed both in life-years and QALYs. Quality-adjusted life years were based on a survey of experts about the health states, and the quality weighting we derived from several multiattribute questionnaires [Quality of Well Being, Health Utilities Index, EuroQol, and Years of Healthy Life; see Patrick and Erickson, (1993)]. The supplementation and all fortification levels were cost saving compared to no program. Fortification at progressively higher levels provided increased savings, with the highest level of savings provided by the highest level of fortification of 0.7 mg of folic acid per 100 mg of cereal grain. Compared with the next level of fortification studied (0.35 mg/100 mg), the highest level of fortification saved \$12,813 per QALY saved. Univariate and multivariate sensitivity analyses were also performed, including best- and worst-case scenarios. None of the sensitivity analyses changed the ordering of the results. Higher levels of fortification provided the greatest cost effectiveness and was cost saving.

The analysis has a number of limitations. The use of the Panel on Cost-Effectiveness in Health and Medicine recommendations regarding the use of QALYs (Gold et al., 1996) underestimates the benefits because productivity costs are not explicitly included. Such losses are considered part of QALYs: thus, including a separate estimate of productivity losses may cause some double accounting. Another limitation is that considerable uncertainty about the risk for masking of B_{12} deficiency remains. Limited longitudinal data were available for children with neural tube defects.

Despite the limitations, the study provided answers to some important questions. The first question, answered positively, was "Is fortifying food with folic acid a cost-saving investment?" The answer to the second question, "Given that food fortification was the preferred strategy, at what level should cereal grain be fortified?" depends on the perspective of the decision maker. The FDA is charged with maintaining a safe food supply. Their primary concern, therefore, is food safety, and consequently the concern about masking of B_{12} deficiency is paramount. Indeed, the preponderance of the debate focused on this issue. The overall economic benefits were therefore a secondary consideration. Ultimately, because of these concerns about safety, a decision was made to recommend fortification at a relatively low level (0.14 mg/100 mg of grain). The cost-utility analysis was important in helping choose a level of fortification that could actually reduce the incidence of neural tube defects while minimizing the risks. Subsequent analyses, which examine fortification at the recommended level along with targeted supplementation, are warranted.

Resource Allocation

Resource allocations can be made on the basis of the results of a CBA or CEA study. In the case of CBA, resources should logically be allocated to those interventions that will provide the largest NPV, assuming that the resources needed are available. The strength of CBA is that such allocations can be made across several different types of interventions, even for very different diseases or conditions.

In the case of CEA-based studies, resources should be allocated to the intervention that provides the lowest cost per unit of health outcome. The problem arises when trying to decide resource allocation between two projects with very different health outcomes. For example, how would you choose between project A, which costs a total of $13 million and provides a CE ratio of $1000 per heart attack prevented; and project B, which costs $7 million and provides a CE ratio of $950 per case of childhood diabetes prevented?

CUA attempts to avoid some of these problems by reducing all interventions to a common health utility outcome such as QALYs. With CUA data, resources are allocated to those projects that cost the least per unit of health utility saved (or save the most per unit of health utility saved). The problem is that this method of resource allocation implies that a QALY saved by preventing heart attacks is equal to a QALY saved by preventing childhood diabetes.

Cost Effectiveness does not Equal Cost Savings

Cost effectiveness does not equal cost savings. Many prevention-orientated interventions result in a net cost for society, rather than a net savings. Tengs et al. (1995) reviewed published literature and evaluated the cost per life saved for 587 health interventions. Approximately 10% of the interventions saved more money than they cost. The median cost per life saved for all interventions was $42,000. Childhood immunizations, many drug treatments, and some prenatal care programs save society money.

Valuing Outcomes: Quality and Other Adjustments

Allocating resources to interventions based solely on economic criteria is fraught with many problems. First, such a method of allocation rarely addresses questions of equity or need. The distribution of health care resources requires a separate study. One method of calculating potential inequalities of health care expenditures involves using the *Gini coefficient* (Fig. 6.2). In Figure 6.2, the 45 degree line represents equal distribution of health care expenditure across all income groups, and the curved line represents a hypothetical actual distribution. The ratio of the areas under the 45 degree line, $A/(A + B)$, gives a coefficient of inequality

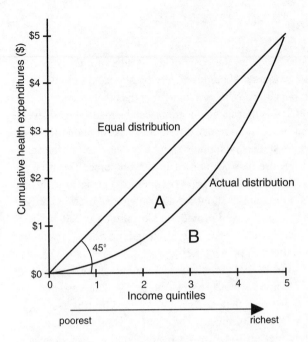

Figure 6.2. A schematic showing how to calculate the Gini coefficient, a measure of equitable distribution.

called the *Gini coefficient*. The larger the coefficient, the greater the inequality. Other methods of considering distribution can be used—the x-axis values could be age groups, or distance from health care centers. The y-axis also can have other values representing health care distribution, such as the number of treatments per person.

One limit to the methodology displayed in Figure 6.2 is that it only defines optimal distribution in terms of complete equality (the 45 degree line). Society may wish to deliberately skew the distribution of health care expenditures. For example, a particular program (e.g., prenatal care) may deliberately be targeted at low-income expectant mothers.

Economic analysis of health interventions has limits. For example, what is the cutoff point or threshold value for cost effectiveness in terms of dollars spent per life saved? Is $50,000 per life saved too much? What about $1.5 million per life saved? And does it matter if the life saved or QALY gained would belong to somebody aged 3 years versus aged 63 years? None of these questions can be answered simply by an economic analysis. An economic evaluation can only provide data for a societal debate as to the value of a given program or set of programs.

References

Ahlbom, A., and S. Norell. *Epidemiology*. Chestnut Hill, MA: Epidemiology Resources, 1990.

Cates, W., and G. D. Williamson. Descriptive epidemiology: analyzing and interpreting surveillance data. In: *Principles and Practice of Public Health Surveillance*, edited by S. M. Teutsch, and E. R. Churchill. New York: Oxford University Press, 1994.

Coughlin, S. S., and T. L. Beauchamp (eds.). *Ethics and Epidemiology*. New York: Oxford University Press, 1996.

Dasbach, E., and S. M. Teutsch. Cost-utility analysis. In: *Prevention Effectiveness: A Guide to Decision Analysis and Economic Evaluation*, edited by A. C. Haddix, S. M. Teutsch, P. A. Shaffer, and D. O. Dunet. New York: Oxford University Press, 1996, pp. 130–142.

Garber, A. M., M. C. Weinstein, G. W. Torrance, and M. S. Kamlet. Theoretical foundations of cost-effectiveness analysis. In: *Cost-Effectiveness in Health and Medicine*, edited by M. R. Gold, J. E. Siegel, L. B. Russell, and M. C. Weinstein. New York: Oxford University Press, 1996, pp. 25–53.

Gill, T. M., and A. R. Feinstein. A critical reappraisal of the quality of quality-of-life measurements. *JAMA* 272:619–626, 1994.

Gold, M. R., J. E. Siegel, L. B. Russell, and M. C. Weinstein (eds.). *Cost-Effectiveness in Health and Medicine*. New York: Oxford University Press, 1996.

Haddix, A. C., S. M. Teutsch, P. A. Shaffer, and D. O. Dunet. *Prevention Effectiveness: A Guide to Decision Analysis and Economic Evaluation*. New York: Oxford University Press, 1996, pp. 172–180.

Kelly, A. E., A. L. Haddix, K. S. Scanlon, et al. Cost-effectiveness of strategies to prevent neural tube defects. In: *Cost-Effectiveness in Health and Medicine*, edited by M. R. Gold, J. E. Siegel, L. B. Russell, and M. C. Weinstein. New York: Oxford University Press, 1996, pp.313–348.

Lipscomb, J., M. C. Weinstein, and G. W. Torrence. Time preference. In *Cost-Effectiveness in Health and Medicine*, edited by M. R. Gold, J. E. Siegel, L. B. Russell, and M. C. Weinstein. New York: Oxford University Press, 1996, pp. 214–235.

Magid, D., B. Schwartz, J. Craft, and J. S. Schwartz. Prevention of Lyme disease after tick bites: a cost-effectiveness analysis. *N. Engl. J. Med.* 327:534–541, 1992.

Murray, C. J. L. Quantifying the burden of disease: the technical basis for disability-adjusted life years. *Bull. World. Health Organ.* 72:429–445, 1994.

National Center or Health Statistics. *Health, United States, 1996–97 and Injury Chartbook*. Hyattsville, MD, 1997.

O'Brien, B. J., D. Helyland, W. S. Richardson, et al. Users' guides to the medical literature. XIII. How to use an article on economic analysis of clinical practice. What are the results and will they help me in caring for my patients. *JAMA* 272:1802–1806, 1997.

Patrick, D. L., and P. Erickson. *Health Status and Health Policy: Allocating Resources to Health Care*. New York: Oxford University Press, 1993.

Rothman, K. J. *Modern Epidemiology*. Boston: Little, Brown & Co., 1986.

Tengs, T. O., M. E. Adams, J. S. Pliskin, et al. Five-hundred life-saving interventions and their cost-effectiveness. *Risk Anal.* 15:369–390, 1995.

Wennberg, J. E., J. L. Freeman, R. M. Shelton, and T. A. Bubolz. Hospital use and mortality among Medicare beneficiaries in Boston and New Haven. *N. Engl. J. Med.* 321: 1168–1173, 1989.

7

Statistical Issues in Developing Guidelines and Policies

ALAN R. HINMAN
ELIZABETH R. ZELL
DIXIE E. SNIDER, JR.

The greater the ignorance the greater the dogmatism.
—Sir William Osler (1849–1919)

Guidelines and policies are increasingly important in improving and standardizing both clinical and public health practice. The rationale for their use ranges from trying to ensure optimal care to trying to contain costs. A federal task force sorted through conflicting evidence on clinical preventive services (e.g., screening, immunization, counseling, and chemoprophylaxis) and developed recommendations for clinicians based on a standardized approach (U.S. Preventive Services Task Force 1996). On the other hand, an expert panel that considered evidence for the use of mammography did not recommend regular mammograms for women under 50 years of age (NIH Consensus statement, 1997).

One result of the increasing emphasis on guidelines has been the development of a scientific body of knowledge about the process of guideline development. Whereas guidelines previously were developed by a variety of means including *consensus development, expert opinion,* and formal *rules of evidence,* increasingly they are being developed by following *explicit protocols.* The Centers for Disease Control and Prevention (CDC) has developed the document "CDC Guidelines: Improving the Quality," which summarizes the important principles of guideline development and making recommendations (CDC, 1996a). The CDC document outlines 13 primary tasks in guideline development:

1. planning and coordinating the process
2. assessing user needs
3. choosing guideline topics
4. selecting guideline panels
5. defining the scope of the guidelines
6. clarifying the method and analytic framework
7. identifying and synthesizing the evidence
8. aiding group interaction and decision making
9. identifying a research agenda
10. updating the guideline
11. writing the guideline
12. obtaining critical reviews and public comment
13. encouraging adoption of the guideline

Another approach has modified these steps in developing clinical practice guidelines, which are "systematically developed statements to assist practitioner and
patient decisions about appropriate health care for specific clinical circumstances" (Agency for Health Care Policy and Research, 1993). Whatever the specific process, the steps followed typically include an explicit description of the
process to be followed, a formal review of evidence (typically concentrating on
articles published in the peer-reviewed literature), categorization of the evidence
reviewed, and an explicit relationship between the level of evidence and the
strength of the recommendation.

Statistical methods play an important role in several phases of guideline development, particularly in assessing the need for the guideline, defining the major
questions to be answered by the guideline, reviewing and analyzing available information, and translating the review of evidence into a guideline. Some of the
techniques associated with these steps are described in the following paragraphs.

Guideline Development

Assessing the Need for the Guideline

This step in guideline development typically involves reviewing evidence concerning the magnitude of the problem, the preventable fraction of the burden of
the condition, and the existence of one or more interventions. Evidence regarding the magnitude of the problem often comes from surveillance information
(see Chapter 3) but also may be developed as a result of specific studies or surveys.

Surveys may be developed on the basis of interviews, reviews of records, physical or laboratory examinations, or some combination of these sources (Levy and

Lemeshow, 1991). Truly *random surveys,* the statistical benchmarks, may be difficult to carry out in practice (due to geographic dispersion or lack of a sampling frame), particularly if they involve face-to-face contact between the surveyor and the subject. In part, to compensate for this difficulty, *cluster surveys* have been devised, in which sampling units may be drawn on the basis of a probability design with each person in the overall study population having a known probability of being selected for the survey at the outset (see Chapter 2). When surveys involve a laboratory component, statistical methods are used for quality control and to ensure replicability of results. We present a case study on lead poisoning to illustrate the importance of laboratory methods and surveys in developing policy.

Because most households have telephones, *telephone surveys* have largely replaced face-to-face interview surveys. Since not all households have telephones, a usual assumption is that households with and without telephones are similar for the characteristics being measured. When this assumption does not hold and inferences are to be made to the entire population, corrections can be made similar to those used to adjust for differences between respondents and nonrespondents (e.g., careful follow-up of a subsample of those without telephones or those who did not respond or independent information from another data source that includes both telephone and nontelephone households). Matching of results from providers (or records) may be carried out to validate the responses given in interviews. We present a case study on immunization to illustrate the value of surveys, surveillance, and evaluation in the development of guidelines.

Assessing the perspectives of the intended users of a guideline is also valuable. Guidelines may have the greatest impact if they meet a specific need (e.g., an emerging health problem, new rules or regulations, requests from constituents or interest groups, new research studies or products, or variation in practice). Empirical confirmation of the need may be obtained from focus groups (Morgan, 1993) or surveys. In addition to assessing the need, these methods can assist with the content and format of the guidelines themselves (e.g., target populations, practice settings, and flexibility of recommendations) (CDC, 1996a).

Defining the Major Questions to Be Answered by the Guidelines

In this step, previously developed consensus or guidelines are examined to find gaps in pertinent information. Because there are often many unanswered questions, the questions may require prioritization based on criteria such as morbidity or economic impact of the problem (or the intervention), conflicting results from available studies (or major controversy), or availability of relevant information. Economic analyses may be of particular relevance in this phase (see Chapter 6).

Reviewing and Analyzing Available Information

This step involves identifying key studies, reviewing such studies, and categorizing the evidence. For the U.S. Preventive Services Task Force (1996), this step involved developing the following hierarchy of evidence: randomized controlled trials, nonrandomized controlled trials, cohort studies, case-control studies, comparisons between time and places, uncontrolled experiments, descriptive studies, and expert opinion.

Because there are often multiple studies of slightly different designs yielding disparate (and sometimes conflicting) results, methods have been developed to synthesize results from several studies. Meta-analysis is an approach that is increasingly being used (Mosteller and Colditz, 1996). *Meta-analysis* is a formal statistical technique for combining the results of different studies to resolve discrepancies among studies and arrive at conclusions about a body of research. This technique is most useful when individual studies have had contradictory results and when study populations have been too small to yield a valid conclusion (Ohlsson, 1994). Meta-analysis primarily has been used to combine the results of randomized trials (Nony et al., 1995). However, meta-analysis of nonexperimental studies also has been done. This is particularly relevant because randomized trials cannot be conducted for many topics of public health interest. For nonexperimental studies, the method is most useful when many studies with low statistical power have been conducted (Petitti, 1994). The major disadvantages of meta-analysis are that (*1*) it is very time consuming and complex and (*2*) it can only be done successfully if several studies that address the research hypothesis have already been completed. The systematic, explicit nature of meta-analysis distinguishes it from qualitative literature reviews. Guidelines for the conduct (Thacker, 1988) and reporting (Rosenthal, 1995) of meta-analysis give explicit procedures for their conduct. There is disagreement about the inclusion of data from unpublished studies, the inclusion of non-English language studies, and quality scoring systems (Petitti, 1994). We present a case study on tuberculosis to illustrate the value of meta-analysis in developing guidelines.

Translating the Review of Evidence into a Guideline

The translation of scientific evidence into a guideline increasingly involves rating the evidence, either qualitatively or quantitatively, and using this as a guide to the strength of the recommendation. For example, the U.S. Preventive Services Task Force (1996) rated evidence using a five-point scale that ranged from "evidence obtained from at least one properly randomized controlled trial" to "opinions of respected authorities, based on clinical experience; descriptive studies and case reports; or reports of expert committees." Recommendations also were made using a five-point scale ranging from "good evidence to support the recommendation" for the use of an intervention, through "insufficient evidence to recommend for or against," to "good evidence to support the recommendation" against using the intervention. The strength of the recommendation generally correlated with the quality of the evidence.

Case Studies

Lead Poisoning Prevention

Lead poisoning can have a severe effect on mental capacity. Recent evidence has indicated that even low body burdens of lead can have a substantial impact on intellectual development (Agency for Toxic Substances and Disease Registry, 1988). In the 1950s, 1960s, and early 1970s, the main source of nonoccupational lead exposure among humans was considered to be lead in paint. Lead from soldered cans was also of concern, and some evidence indicated that lead in gasoline might be an important source of exposure.

In 1975, as part of its regulatory efforts for air pollutants, the Environmental Protection Agency (EPA) began requiring catalytic converters on new cars. To work properly, catalytic converters required unleaded gasoline. As a result, starting in 1975, the amount of unleaded gasoline used in the United States gradually began to increase—thus causing the amount of total lead used in gasoline to decline. Environmental modeling based on the available data projected that reducing lead in gasoline would have only a slight effect on the blood lead levels of persons living in the United States. Lead is an inexpensive octane booster, and increasing the amount of lead in leaded gasoline would reduce the cost of producing higher octane leaded gasoline. In 1981, based on these modeling predictions, EPA put forth a proposal to *increase* the amount of lead in leaded gasoline.

Concerned that the adoption of this policy would have an adverse effect on health, researchers from the Department of Health and Human Services (DHHS) analyzed data from the 1976–1980 National Health and Nutrition Examination Survey (NHANES II). The analysis demonstrated a significant decline in mean blood lead levels during the course of the examination cycle (Annest et al., 1983). The magnitude of the decline in blood lead levels resulting from the decrease in lead in gasoline was approximately tenfold greater than had been predicted by the environmental modeling and closely paralleled the decrease in lead used in gasoline (Fig. 7.1). The result of these analyses was the dominant factor that caused the EPA to reverse its previous proposal to increase the lead in leaded gasoline and instead adopt regulations that more rapidly removed lead from all gasoline.

NHANES is a periodic survey carried out by the CDC's National Center for Health Statistics (NCHS) (U.S. Department of Health and Human Services, 1981). It uses a stratified, multistage, probability-based cluster design of the civilian noninstitutionalized population and can be designed to oversample spe-

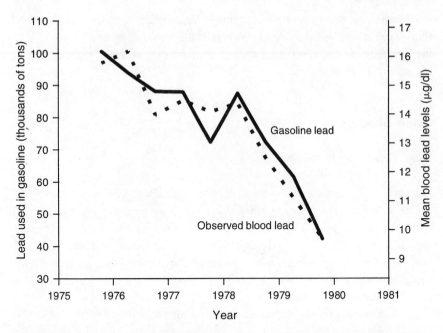

Figure 7.1. Relationship between lead in gasoline and mean blood lead levels: NHANES II, 1976–1980.

cific population groups. For example, during 1982–1984, a special survey was carried out of Mexican-Americans living in the southwest United States (Hispanic NHANES). In the surveys, a standardized questionnaire is administered by an interviewer through a household visit. Physical examinations are carried out at a mobile examination center, and for children, lead levels from venous blood specimens are measured. By the time NHANES III had been implemented (1988–1991), new national estimates of blood lead levels were available. By this time, 99.8% of lead in gasoline in the United States had been removed, and blood lead levels in the U.S. population had decreased by 78%. Further analysis of the NHANES III data indicated that particular groups of children were at higher risk of lead poisoning, including children who live in central cities, children in families of lower income, and black or Mexican-American children (Fig. 7.2). These findings indicate that there are remaining sources of lead exposure (e.g., in soil and in paint that has already been applied) that must be dealt with before lead poisoning is eliminated as a cause of mental retardation in this country. They also underscore the multifactorial nature of environmental health problems.

U.S. Immunization Policy

The elimination of vaccine-preventable diseases is a priority of public health activities throughout the world. Beginning in 1957, a set of questions about vac-

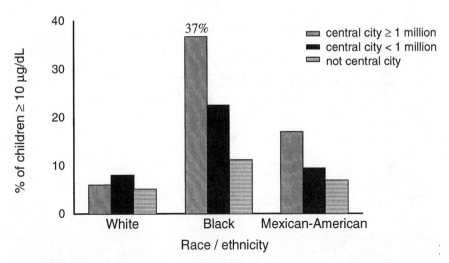

Figure 7.2. Percent of children aged 1–5 years with blood lead ≥ 10 μg/dL by residence and race/ethnicity (NHANES III 1988–91).

cination status was added to the ongoing Current Population Survey carried out by the Bureau of the Census (Sirken and Brenner, 1960; Sirken, 1962; Morris, 1964). Data from this U.S. Immunization Survey (USIS) allowed estimates of vaccination coverage at the national level by age, race, urban/rural residence, and socioeconomic status, although state-specific estimates could not be made (Eddins et al., 1995). Figure 7.3 demonstrates the trends in vaccination levels for 1967–1995.

In the 1970s, approximately 20 million U.S. children lacked at least one dose of one vaccine to be fully vaccinated, and the incidence of measles increased (Hinman, 1979). As a result, in April 1977, a national childhood immunization initiative was announced with two goals: attainment of immunization levels of 90% for the nation's children by October 1979 and establishment of a permanent system to provide comprehensive immunization services to the 3 million children born in America each year. A broad-based program was undertaken involving increased federal support for immunizations, increased involvement of volunteers in all aspects of immunization activities, increased public awareness/public education activities, and increased cooperation between governmental activities. Federal immunization grant funds to state health departments increased dramatically. Efforts were expanded to enact school immunization requirements in states that did not have them and to enforce those already in existence. As a result of these efforts, all 50 states soon had, and were enforcing, school entry laws. Since 1981, 95% or more of children entering school have records documenting receipt of required vaccinations. Given these levels, even with lower levels in preschoolers, the overall vaccination level in children of all ages in this country is 90% or greater.

In the late 1980s, outbreaks of measles in preschool children indicated that

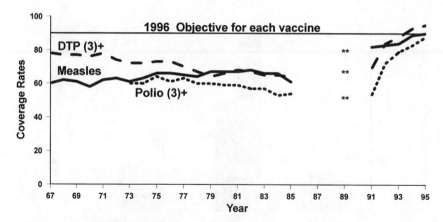

Figure 7.3. Vaccine-specific coverage rates among U.S. 2-Year-Olds, 1967–1995 (2-year-olds defined as 24–35 months for 1967–1985 and 19–35 months for 1991–1995). **Funding for surveys eliminated 1986–1990. [From USIS (1967–1985) and NHIS (1991–1993), National Immunization Survey, 1994–1995.]

high levels of vaccination at school entry did not ensure that these children were immunized on time (Fig. 7.4) (Zell et al., 1994). In 1991, a national effort was launched to raise vaccination levels by the year 2000 so that 90% or more of the nation's children would routinely complete the basic series of vaccinations by their second birthday. This marked a turning point, and, with President Clinton's 1993 announcement of a new childhood immunization initiative, a major infusion of funds was brought to bear on vaccinating infants and young children.

To identify states and cities that were having particular problems vaccinating children, the National Immunization Survey (NIS) was developed (CDC, 1997) to provide national, state, and selected urban area estimates of vaccination coverage levels among children aged 19–35 months. The NIS uses a two-phase sample design: the first phase employs a quarterly random sample of telephone numbers for each survey area and includes administration of a screening questionnaire to respondents aged 18 years or older to locate households with one or more children aged 19–35 months. In the second phase, vaccination information is requested from health care providers of children in surveyed households. Standard two-phase estimation procedures were used to estimate vaccination coverage for each surveyed area. Estimates were adjusted for nonresponse using birth data adjusted for infant mortality and migration to create a weighted sample representative of children aged 19–35 months in the United States. In addition, adjustments were made for exclusion of households without a telephone, because children in households without telephones are less likely to be vaccinated than children in households with telephones (Zell et al., 1996).

The NIS determined that, among children born during February 1992 through May 1994 who were aged 19–35 months (median age: 27 months) at the time of

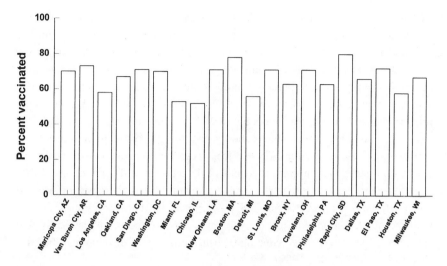

Figure 7.4. Percent of children vaccinated with MMR by 24 months: retrospective school entrant surveys, 1991–1992.

the survey, the estimated vaccination coverage was 95% for three or more doses of diphtheria and tetanus toxoids and pertussis (*DTP*) vaccine, 92% for three or more doses of *Haemophilus influenzae* type b (*Hib*) vaccine, 88% for three or more doses of poliovirus vaccine, and 90% for one dose of measles-containing vaccine [typically measles, mumps, and rubella (*MMR*) vaccine]. Estimated vaccination coverage was 76% (95% confidence interval ± 1.0%) for receipt of at least four doses of DTP, three doses of poliovirus vaccine, and one dose of MMR (4:3:1 series). The lower overall coverage for the series compared with coverage for individual vaccination was accounted for primarily by low coverage with the fourth dose of DTP (79%).

To assess the validity of estimates from the NIS, findings were compared with coverage estimates from the National Health Interview Survey, which had been supplemented with provider information in the same manner as the NIS during 1994. The estimated series complete coverage levels were similar in the two surveys, and the coverage levels for individual vaccines were nearly identical.

Meta-analysis, BCG Vaccine, and Tuberculosis Prevention

Early in the twentieth century, the French researchers Calmette and Guérin developed a vaccine using attenuated *Mycobacterium bovis* organisms which they hoped would prevent tuberculosis (TB) in persons who received the vaccine (Fine, 1988). The vaccine, called bacille Calmette-Guérin (BCG), was first used in humans in 1921 and has since gained wide acceptance throughout the world.

Almost since the introduction of BCG, however, there has been disagreement about its efficacy, with published studies reporting vaccine efficacy as high as 80% and as low as − 57% (i.e., vaccinees were more likely to get TB than persons who did not receive vaccine) (Clemens et al., 1983). Questions were raised about the methodology and interpretation of these studies, and attitudes towards BCG achieved near-religious fervor in some discussions. In the United States, three primary reasons were given for not using BCG vaccine: doubts about its efficacy, the low risk of TB in this country, and the fact that BCG vaccination resulted in conversion of the tuberculin skin test from negative to positive. Tuberculin test conversion is the most important means of detecting new TB infections. Tuberculin testing of persons at high risk, followed by preventive therapy for those with positive tests, is a cornerstone of U.S. tuberculosis prevention programs. Persons with recent tuberculin skin test conversion can be treated prophylactically with antituberculosis drugs, thus reducing their lifetime risk of developing tuberculosis by 70%–90% (CDC, 1989).

A multisponsored, large-scale, placebo-controlled field trial of BCG vaccine was carried out in India in the 1970s in an attempt to provide a definitive answer to the question of BCG efficacy. The trial did not show efficacy of BCG in protecting adults against tuberculosis (Baily et al., 1980). However, several mitigating factors were identified that made it impossible to view the results as definitive. Consequently, the debate about the use of BCG continued and national policies remained unchanged.

In the United States, reported tuberculosis incidence declined steadily at an annual rate of 3%–5% starting in 1953 when TB became reportable on a national level, and continuing until the mid-1980s when the incidence reached a plateau and then began to increase. Several factors were cited as being responsible for the increased incidence: deterioration of the public health infrastructure; increased immigration from countries with high prevalence of TB; the human immunodeficiency virus (HIV) epidemic; and outbreaks of TB in hospitals, prisons, and other congregative settings (Ellner et al., 1993). Many of these outbreaks involved multidrug-resistant (MDR) organisms, raising new questions about the use of BCG vaccine in the United States, particularly among health care workers.

The Public Health Service Advisory Committee on Immunization Practices (ACIP) and the Advisory Committee for the Elimination of Tuberculosis (ACET), in consultation with the Hospital Infection Control Practices Advisory Committee (HICPAC), jointly addressed the issue of BCG vaccination. In the absence of new data concerning efficacy, it was determined that a meta-analysis of existing information could be useful in revising existing guidelines. Consequently, such an analysis was commissioned (Colditz et al., 1994). Independently, a second meta-analysis was conducted (Rodrigues et al., 1993).

In the particular case of BCG vaccination, publication bias was not felt to be a major problem because use of the vaccine has been controversial since it was first introduced in the 1920s, probably resulting in the publication of virtually all studies. In addition, in one of the meta-analyses, the authors repeated the analysis using the results of the 13 prospective trials included in the base analysis, but adding 20 hypothetical trials, each equivalent in size to the single largest trial and each showing that no benefit was gained from BCG vaccination. The efficacy remained statistically significant.

One meta-analysis (Colditz et al., 1994) indicated a significant positive protective effect of BCG vaccine in protecting against all forms of TB (combined), miliary TB, TB meningitis, and death from TB. More than 80% of the variance among study results could be explained by the incidence of TB in the population and by the distance of the study site from the equator, with studies conducted nearer the equator showing lower protection. The overall efficacy was estimated to be 50%, and efficacy against more severe disease was thought to be higher. The design and reporting of the limited number of studies of the efficacy of BCG vaccination in protecting health care workers precluded a formal meta-analysis, but the reviewers determined that the studies suggested that vaccination with BCG is effective in reducing the incidence of tuberculosis among health care workers (Brewer and Colditz, 1995).

Another meta-analysis found the protective effect of BCG against pulmonary disease to be heterogeneous and the authors elected not to calculate a summary measure of overall protection (Colditz et al., 1994). However, the summary protective effect against miliary or meningeal TB was 86% in randomized controlled trials and 75% in case-control studies.

In balancing the results of these meta-analyses with the overall low risk of TB in the United States and the efficacy of properly applied TB prevention and control techniques, ACIP and ACET did not feel that widespread use of BCG was warranted in the United States (CDC, 1996b). However, they did recommend consideration of its use in infants or children if exposed continually to an untreated or ineffectively treated patient with infectious pulmonary TB. For health care workers, they recommended consideration of BCG vaccination on an individual basis in settings where (*1*) a high percentage of TB patients are infected with MDR strains, (*2*) transmission is considered likely, and (*3*) comprehensive TB infection-control precautions have been implemented and have not been successful.

Thus, in this situation, the statistical techniques provided an improved estimate of the efficacy of BCG vaccination. Although the data did not indicate a compelling argument for its widespread use given the epidemiological circumstances in the United States, they did support its limited use in infants, children, and health care workers under specific conditions.

Conclusion

The previously described examples demonstrate some of the ways statistical techniques can be used in developing public health guidelines and policies. In the case of lead in gasoline, having data from a valid statistical sample of the U.S. population was decisive in preventing a policy change that could have increased lead poisoning. The example of immunization surveys indicates the importance of ongoing surveys in guiding program policies and actions. The BCG example illustrates how meta-analysis can be useful in approaching highly controversial subjects with studies yielding markedly contrasting results. In addition to demonstrating the importance of statistical approaches in policy development, the examples also demonstrate the critical role of human judgment in assessing the meaning of data, as well as their statistical significance.

References

Agency for Health Care Policy and Research. *Clinical Practice Guideline Development. AHCPR Program Note.* Washington, DC: United States Department of Health and Human Services, August 1993.

Agency for Toxic Substances and Disease Registry. *The Nature and Extent of Lead Poisoning in Children in the United States: A Report to Congress.* Atlanta, GA: United States Department of Health and Human Services, Public Health Service, 1988.

Annest, J. I., J. L. Pirkle, D. Makuc, J. W. Neese, D. D. Bayse, and M. G. Kovar. Chronological trend in blood lead levels between 1976 and 1980. *N. Engl. J. Med.* 308: 1373–1377, 1983.

Baily, G.V. J., R. Narain, S. Mayurnath, R. S. Vallishayee, and J. Guld. Trial of BCG vaccines in south India for tuberculosis prevention: tuberculosis prevention trial, Madras. *Indian J. Med. Res.* 72(Suppl.)S1–S74, 1980.

Brewer, T. F., and G. A. Colditz. Bacille Calmette-Guérin vaccination for the prevention of tuberculosis in healthcare workers. *Clin. Infect. Dis.* 20:136–142, 1995.

Centers for Disease Control. A strategic plan for the elimination of tuberculosis in the United States. *MMWR Morb. Mortal. Wkly. Rep.* 38(Suppl. 3);S1–S25, 1989.

Centers for Disease Control and Prevention. *CDC Guidelines: Improving the Quality.* Atlanta, GA: Centers for Disease Control and Prevention, 1996a.

Centers for Disease Control and Prevention. The role of BCG vaccine in the prevention and control of tuberculosis in the United States: a joint statement by the Advisory Council for the Elimination of Tuberculosis and the Advisory Committee on Immunization Practices. *MMWR Morb. Mortal. Wkly. Rep.* 45(RR-4):1–18, 1996b.

Centers for Disease Control and Prevention. National, state, and urban area vaccination coverage levels among children aged 19–35 months—United States, January–December 1995. *MMWR Morb. Mortal. Wkly. Rep.* 46:176–182, 1997.

Clemens, J. D., J. J. H. Chuong, and A. R. Feinstein. The BCG controversy: a methodological and statistical reappraisal. *JAMA* 249:2362–2369, 1983.

Colditz, G. A., T. F. Brewer, C. S. Berkey, et al. Efficacy of BCG vaccine in the prevention of tuberculosis: meta-analysis of the published literature. *JAMA* 271:698–702, 1994.

Eddins, D. L., B. I. Sirotkin, P. Holmgreen, and S. Russell. *Assessment and Validation of*

Immunization Status in the U.S. Proceedings of the 20th Immunization Conference, May 6–9, 1985. Atlanta, GA: Centers for Disease Control and Prevention, 1995.

Ellner, J. J., A. R. Hinman, S. W. Dooley, et al. Tuberculosis symposium: emerging problems and promise. *J. Infect. Dis.* 168:537–551, 1993.

Fine, P. E. BCG vaccination against tuberculosis and leprosy. *Br. Med. Bull.* 44:691–703, 1988.

Hinman, A. R. A new U.S. initiative in childhood immunization. *B. Pan. Am. Health Organ.* 13:169–176, 1979.

Levy, P. S., and S. Lemeshow. *Sampling of Populations: Methods and Applications.* New York: John Wiley & Sons, 1991.

Morris, L. Further analysis of national participation in the inactivated poliomyelitis vaccination program, 1955–61. *Public Health Rep.* 79:469–480, 1964.

Morgan, D. L., R. A. Krueger, and J. A. King. *Focus Group Kit,* Vols. 1–6. Thousand Oaks, CA: Sage, 1997.

Mosteller, F., and F. A. Colditz. Understanding research synthesis (meta-analysis). *Ann. Rev. Public Health* 17:1–23, 1996.

NIH Consensus Statement. Breast Cancer Screening for Women, ages 40–49. *NIH Consensus Statement* Jan 21:1–35, 1997.

Nony, P., M., M. Cucherat, C. Haugh, and J. P. Boissel. Critical reading of the meta-analysis of clinical trials. *Therapie* 50:339–351, 1995.

Ohlsson, A. Systematic reviews-theory and practice. *Scand. J. Clin. Lab. Invest.* 219 (Suppl.):S25–S32, 1994.

Pettiti, D. B. *Meta-analysis, Decision Analysis, and Cost-effectiveness Analysis.* New York: Oxford University Press, 1994.

Rodrigues, L. C., V. K. Diwan, and J. G. Wheeler. Protective effect of BCG against tuberculous meningitis and miliary tuberculosis: a meta-analysis. *Int. J. Epidemiol.* 22: 1154–1158, 1993.

Rosenthal, R. Writing meta-analytic reviews. *Psychol. Bull.* 118:183–192, 1995.

Sirken, M. G. National participation trends, 1955–1961 in the poliomyelitis vaccination program. *Public Health Rep.* 77:661–670, 1962.

Sirken, M. G., and B. Brenner. *Population Characteristics and Participation in the Poliomyelitis Vaccination Program.* Washington, DC: U.S. Government Printing Office, PHS Publication No. 723, Public Health Monograph No. 61, 1960.

Thacker, S. B. Meta-analysis: a quantitative approach to research integration. *JAMA* 259(11):1685–1689, 1988.

U.S. Department of Health and Human Services. *Vital and Health Statistics: Data Systems of the National Center for Health Statistics.* Washington, DC: U.S. Department of Health and Human Services Publication, DHHS Publication No. (PHS) 82–1318, 1981.

U.S. Preventive Services Task Force. *Guide to Clinical Preventive Services,* 2nd ed. Baltimore, MD: Williams & Wilkins, 1996.

Zell, E. R., V. Dietz, J. Stevenson, S. Cochi, and R. H. Bruce. Low vaccination levels of U.S. preschool and school-age children—retrospective assessments of vaccination coverage, 1991–1992. *JAMA* 271:833–839, 1994.

Zell, E. R., T. M. Ezzati-Rice, J. T. Massey, and J. M. Brick. Response errors associated with household reports of immunizations—analysis of subgroup differences. *Proceedings of the Section of Survey Research Methods.* Alexandria VA: American Statistical Association, 1996.

8

Implementing and Managing Programs

EDUARDO J. SIMOES
ROSS C. BROWNSON

Learn my son with how little wisdom the world is governed.
—Pope Julius, III (1487–1555)

Managers in public health settings are increasingly called upon to develop, implement, and evaluate programs, with the goal of demonstrating and replicating those that are effective. A *public health program* can be defined as a structured intervention or policy change aimed to improve the health of the total population or a subpopulation at particularly high risk. Public health programs depend on a variety of inputs and outputs and often have short-term, intermediate, and long-term objectives. For example, programs such as the American Stop Smoking Study for Cancer Prevention (ASSIST) or Initiatives to Mobilize for the Prevention and Control of Tobacco Use (IMPACT) are designed to mobilize coalitions to enhance tobacco control policies at the city, county, and state levels (Siegfried, 1991; CDC, 1996). A short-term objective of these programs is to develop viable coalitions; an intermediate objective is to enact effective policies; and a longer-term objective is to decrease tobacco use and thus decrease death and disability caused by tobacco use.

There are numerous impediments to the development, implementation, and maintenance of effective programs in public health agencies. First, program implementation is not always based on scientific evidence. Second, public health professionals often are in a position of reacting to crises, which makes proactive program planning and long-term commitment to a program difficult. Third, effective program development is complex and depends on multiple disciplines and skills.

This chapter is intended to help program managers increase the effectiveness

165

of their programs. It includes conceptual issues for implementing and monitoring programs, statistical issues, a case study to illustrate key points, and suggestions for further research.

CONCEPTUAL FRAMEWORKS

Over the past few decades, numerous *health planning models* have been proposed to help public health professionals develop more systematic approaches to health program implementation and management. Examples of these models include (*1*) *p*redisposing, *r*einforcing, and *e*nabling *c*onstructs in *e*ducational/*e*nvironmental *d*iagnosis and *e*valuation (PRECEDE) (*2*) *p*olicy, *r*egulatory, and *o*rganizational *c*onstructs in *e*ducational and *e*nvironmental *d*evelopment (PROCEED) (Green and Kreuter, 1991); (*3*) the *p*lanned *a*pproach *t*o *c*ommunity *h*ealth (PATCH) (CDC, 1992), and (*4*) *m*ultilevel *a*pproach *t*o *c*ommunity *h*ealth (MATCH) (Simons-Morton et al., 1988). A discussion of the various models is beyond the scope of this chapter. However, many of the common elements of these approaches are shown in Figure 8.1. All of the models begin with a formal needs assessment and proceed to policy formulation (including goal setting), program planning, and implementation. Evaluation is a critical part of the process because it helps to reformulate the program along the way and determines the effectiveness of the program when completed. The following sections discuss several tools that can be assets for program managers who are responsible for planning and implementing programs.

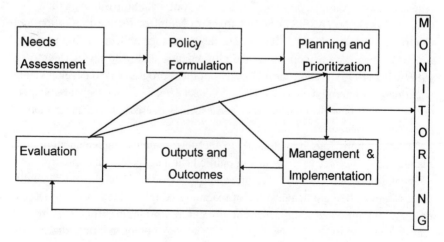

Figure 8.1 Interrelationships between various components of public health program development. [From Holland, WW, 1983.]

Continuous Quality Improvement

The processes of *continuous quality improvement (CQI)* and *total quality management (TQM)* have been frequently utilized in the health care arena in recent years. As is often the case in the literature, CQI and TQM will be used synonymously in this chapter. A recent survey of 3303 hospitals revealed that 69% had actively begun to implement the basic components of CQI (Barsness et al., 1993). CQI has been utilized largely in response to health reform initiatives and the growth of managed care. For health care organizations, the major goal of CQI is to maintain and improve quality in health care while controlling increases in cost (Shortell et al., 1995b). Shortell et al. (1995a) have described the "pyramid" of CQI (Fig. 8.2). Key elements are:

cultural—the underlying beliefs, values, norms and behaviors of the organization

technical—the extent to which employees have received training in CQI tools (e.g., cause-and-effect diagrams and statistical process control charts)

strategic—the extent to which the organization's CQI efforts are focused on key strategic initiatives and on an overall strategic plan

structural—specific organizational entities (e.g., coordinating committees, work groups, and reporting/accountability mechanisms)

CQI is a participative, systematic approach to program planning and implementation (Kaluzny et al., 1992). A central tenet of CQI is that quality is made by processes, not by people (Deming, 1960; Deming, 1986). The key elements of CQI include (*1*) satisfying customers' expectations, (*2*) identifying problems, (*3*) building commitment, and (*4*) promoting open decision making. Berwick et al. (1991) have defined ten basic principles of CQI (Table 8.1). Modern CQI uses the

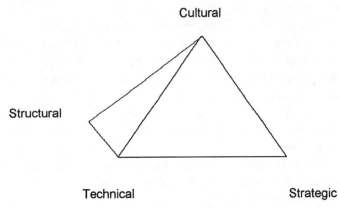

Figure 8.2 The pyramid of continuous quality improvement. [From Shortell et al., 1995b.].

Table 8.1 Ten Basic Principles of Continuous Quality Improvement*

1. Productive work is accomplished through processes.
2. Sound customer-supplier relationships are absolutely necessary for sound quality management.
3. The main source of quality defects is problems in the process.
4. Poor quality is costly.
5. Understanding the variability of processes is a key to improving quality.
6. Quality control should focus on the most vital processes.
7. The modern approach to quality is thoroughly grounded in scientific and statistical thinking.
8. Total employee involvement is critical.
9. New organizational structures can help achieve quality improvement.
10. Quality management employs three basic, closely related interrelated activities: quality planning, quality control, and quality improvement.

*From Berwick et al., 1991.

scientific method to understand and improve processes and relies heavily on the use of quality improvement "teams" to define processes and solutions (Berwick et al., 1991). The notion of *"statistical quality control"* has grown along with the CQI movement. Statistical quality control often relates to "process control," or the monitoring of a routine operating process (Hamaker et al., 1978). Process control can be used in diverse settings (e.g., learning experiments, stock markets, and computer data preparation). Process control involves the monitoring of a given process with an inspection scheme. Procedures can then be put in place for automatically detecting departures from targets and making adjustments (Box and Jenkins, 1962).

CQI approaches have intrinsic appeal for use in the field of public health because of the scientific basis of public health (e.g., through epidemiological research) and the multidisciplinary nature of public health. Readers are referred elsewhere (Berwick et al., 1991; McLaughlin and Kaluzny, 1994) for detailed discussions of CQI and its applications in health care. CQI encompasses an array of managerial issues including leadership, governance, and human resources management (Arrington et al., 1995; Haddock et al., 1995).

Although CQI has been described as a major managerial innovation for public health agencies, the application of CQI principles in public health agencies has been extremely limited (Kaluzny et al., 1992). In part, the breadth of public health makes CQI applications more difficult. For example, a key aspect of CQI is the improvement of customer satisfaction. Health care organizations have both internal and external customers. The internal customer is the health care worker, whereas the external customer is the person seeking health care or the patient (Berwick et al., 1991). However, because health departments are responsible for the health of the entire population, the external customer is more diffuse. In recent years, the notion of "customer-driven government" has grown in prominence (Osborne and Gaebler, 1992).

Traditional approaches to managing public health programs and CQI methods are not mutually exclusive. However, Kaluzny et al. (1992) have highlighted differences between the two approaches that should be considered (Table 8.2). Public health applications of CQI often involve a locus shift from the institution to the community. A series of "action steps" may be useful in achieving this shift to a wider population focus (Table 8.3). Health indicators can inform several of these steps and are discussed in detail later in this chapter.

The recently developed Assessment Protocol for Excellence in Public Health (APEX-PH) may be a useful tool for public health practitioners who wish to address some of the issues using a CQI model. APEX-PH is a community process for setting health status goals and program objectives (National Association of County Health Officials, 1991). It is a process to assist local health departments in assessing and improving their organization and in working with the local community to assess and improve community health status (Oberle et al., 1994). The workbook format of APEX-PH is among the earliest approaches to systematic assessment of organizational factors in relation to the community being served.

Priority Setting and Evaluation

Establishing public health and health care priorities in an era of limited resources is a demanding task. Uses of quantitative approaches and systematic evaluation can make important contributions to priority setting.

Priority Setting

Public health leaders began to formulate concrete public health objectives as a basis for action during the post–World War II era. This was a clear shift from earlier efforts as emphasis was increasingly placed on quantifiable objectives and ex-

Table 8.2. Comparisons of the Traditional Management Model with the Continuous Quality Improvement (CQI)*

Traditional Model	CQI Model
Legal or professional authority	Collective or managerial responsibility
Specialized accountability	Process accountability
Administrative authority	Participation
Meeting standards	Meeting process and performance expectations
Longer planning horizon	Shorter planning horizon
Quality assurance	Continuous improvement

*From Kaluzny et al., 1992.

Table 8.3 Action Steps for Moving Continuous Quality Improvement (CQI) from Institutional to Community-Based Application*

Be cautious in implementing a CQI infrastructure that may have worked in intraorganizational initiatives.
Achieve the commitment of top management to community-based needs assessment.
Develop long-run strategic objectives, but also set short-term measurable objectives.
Select topics to utilize network participants who are ready for a common quality improvement approach to specific objectives, capitalizing on "small wins."
Emphasize data feedback and improved insight.
Avoid "religious" wars—to not try to convert adherents to other approaches to one's version of the "best" approach.
Remember that time is a perishable commodity.
Use "double-loop" learning—participating organizations should understand both the basic definitions of CQI and the underlying assumptions.
Build the network of organizations carefully.
Recognize initial efforts as a coalition arrangement.
Consider the synergistic effects of the community and individual.
Establish capitation and other financial arrangements.
Recognize the liability of trade-offs–a shift from acute care to prevention may shift the power structure.
Reemphasize the cost-quality relationships.

*From Kaluzny et al., 1995.

plicit time limits (Breslow, 1990). Measuring progress toward explicit goals has become an essential feature of priority setting.

Recently, the U.S. Public Health Service established three overarching health goals for the year 2000: (*1*) increase the span of healthy life for Americans; (*2*) reduce health disparities among Americans; and (*3*) achieve access to preventive services for all Americans (U.S. Department of Health and Human Services, 1990). To achieve these three goals, a comprehensive set of 300 main health objectives was established in 22 priority areas. A total of 223 special populations are targeted (e.g., persons with low incomes, persons with disabilities, or those who are members of a racial/ethnic minority group). The core of the year 2000 objectives is based on decades of epidemiological research showing modifiable risk factors that could substantially influence the disease burden in the United States (U.S. Department of Health and Human Services, 1990). Progress toward the year 2000 objectives is being measured in annual reports (National Center for Health Statistics 1996a). These reports place each objective into one of four categories: (*1*) met or progress made, (*2*) moved away from target, (*3*) mixed or no change, and (*4*) cannot assess. Establishment of national, quantifiable objectives has stimulated state and local efforts in program planning, implementation, and evaluation. For example, an estimated 70% of all 3000 U.S. local health agencies have used Healthy People 2000 objectives (National Association of County and City Health Officials, 1995). Public health indicators are important features of the objective-setting process and will be discussed in detail later in this chapter (see Public Health Indicators).

Program Evaluation

The evaluation of the effects of public health programs on the health of the population is one of the ten practices defined as a core function of public health (Dyal, 1995). Likewise, assessing the health needs of the community is an integral part of these core functions (Institute of Medicine, 1988; Dyal, 1991). In the past 5 years, some researchers have proposed clear and scientific protocols to appraise performance of these core functions in public health agencies (Miller et al., 1994; Turnock et al., 1994).

As shown in Figure 8.1, evaluation is one of the key components of program implementation and management. The most fundamental question in program evaluation is: Did the program accomplish its stated objectives? In other words, was the program effective? Other chapters in this book address economic evaluation (see Chapter 6) and outcome evaluation (see Chapter 9). A brief overview of evaluation is provided in this chapter, with primary emphasis on process and impact evaluation.

Types of Evaluation

The various types of evaluation provide information that may be used by program managers, policy makers, and planners. Green and Lewis (1986) defined program evaluation in three categories based on the type of decision making: *diagnostic, formative,* and *summative.* Diagnostic evaluation is part of needs assessment and attempts to determine which persons or group of persons are at highest risk for a particular health condition. Formative evaluation is concerned with identifying any needed adjustments in the process of implementing a program. Therefore, such evaluation usually is conducted midway during program implementation. Summative evaluation is usually carried out after program completion, aiming to identify needed modifications before program continuation or enactment of a similar program elsewhere.

In another classification scheme for program evaluation, Green and Kreuter (1991) defined evaluation in three distinct levels: *process, impact,* and *outcome.* Process evaluation is concerned with asking the questions: What was done? To whom, and how? Impact evaluation is concerned with the questions: What results were obtained after program activity was implemented? What are the most immediate outputs of program implementation and how many were generated? Finally, outcome evaluation is concerned with identifying the changes in target outcomes such as mortality, morbidity, disability, and quality of life. A systems approach will enable one to conceptualize the different levels of a health program, evaluation inclusive, as a continuous cycle (Figure 8.1).

Generally, the following terms are used interchangeably: *needs assessment* and *diagnostic evaluation; process* and *formative evaluation*; and *impact, outcome,* and *summative evaluation* (Green and Lewis, 1986). At times, a distinction is made between process and formative evaluation. The former is limited to monitoring the implementation of a program, the latter to a pilot study with immediate feedback on process and impact that can be used for revision of program components, instruments, and data collection procedures.

Public Health Indicators

The need for *public health indicators* is a common feature of establishing CQI, setting program priorities, evaluating programs, analyzing cost effectiveness, and assessing public health agencies' performance. Strategic planning efforts at the community level can directly benefit from the use of health indicators (e.g., years of potential life lost and excess costs of morbidity and mortality).

Indicators are markers of a given situation, or reflections of that situation. They are usually defined as variables that help to measure change (WHO, 1981a). Health indicators are measures of the extent to which targets in health programs are being reached. Indicators are not numerical targets in themselves and should not be confused with objectives and targets, which tend to be more specific and quantifiable according to some scale or time.

Indicators can help to stimulate public health action. By providing a benchmark, indicators can help program managers and policymakers reformulate existing strategies. Public health indicators can be considered "horizontal" (e.g., comparing rates or services among the states or provinces within a country) or "vertical" (e.g., comparing rates or services at the local, state, or federal level). Health indicators also can be classified according to the type of program (e.g., health services delivery vs. health promotion and education), scope of program objectives (e.g., tobacco control vs. sexually transmitted diseases), or type of evaluation (e.g., process vs. outcome). For example, for the World Health Organization (WHO), indicators of progress towards year 2000 objectives were comprehensive and included major areas of health policy, health-related social and economic factors, provision of health care, and health status (Table 8.4).

The indicators of progress toward Health for All 2000 (WHO, 1981b) were comprehensive in scope because the WHO-HFA is a comprehensive strategy to achieve levels of health that enable persons to lead socially and economically productive lives. They were based on comparisons among countries and among regions within a country. In addition, they were created with the assumption that most WHO-HFA participating countries had some form of comprehensive na-

Table 8.4 Examples of Indicators Related to Health within Four Major Areas*

Major Area	Indicator
Health policy	Political commitment to health for all
	Resource allocation
	The degree of equity of distribution of health resources
	Community involvement in attaining health for all
	Organizational framework and managerial process
Social and economic	Rate of population increase
	Gross national product and gross domestic product
	Income distribution
	Work conditions
	Adult literacy rate
	Housing
	Food availability
Provision of health care	Coverage by primary health care
	Coverage by referral system
Health status	Nutritional status and psychosocial development of children
	Infant mortality rate
	Child mortality rate (aged 1–4 years)
	Life expectancy at birth or other specific ages
	Maternal mortality rate

From World Health Organization, 1981b.

tional health services. At present, health resources are not shared equally by all persons, resulting in significant gaps in health status in many countries. The WHO-HFA year 2000 indicators were also constructed to reflect international differences in the progress toward correcting this imbalance in health resource distributions within a country. Finally, a WHO set of health indicators was designed for use among all countries including those with either incipient policies regarding a specific health issue or no policies at all. Measuring political commitment was a significant first step in this strategy.

Similarly, the U.S. Centers for Disease Control and Prevention (CDC) developed a consensus set of 18 health status indicators in 1991 (Table 8.5). A recent survey of all U.S. state health departments gathered information on which of these indicators is actually being monitored in each state (Zucconi and Carson, 1994). The survey found that mortality indicators were monitored in nearly all states, except for work-related deaths, which were tracked in 75.5% of states. Most other indicators in Table 8.5 were monitored at high levels with the exceptions of poor air quality (tracked in 46.9% of states) and childhood poverty (tracked in 58.8% of states). At the county and state levels, these indicators have proven valuable in measuring progress in disease prevention and health promotion (Sutocky et al., 1996).

Another type of indicator that has been primarily used in evaluation of the delivery and quality of health care is the *performance indicator.* A performance indicator has been defined as an "interrelated set of process and/or outcome mea-

Table 8.5 The Centers for Disease Control and Prevention's Consensus Set of Health Status Indicators*

1. Race-ethnicity—specific infant mortality rate
2. Motor vehicle crash death rate
3. Work-related injury death rate
4. Suicide rate
5. Lung cancer death rate
6. Breast cancer death rate
7. Cardiovascular disease death rate
8. Homicide rate
9. All-cause mortality rate
10. AIDS incidence
11. Measles incidence
12. Tuberculosis incidence
13. Syphilis incidence
14. Incidence of low birth weight
15. Births among adolescents
16. Prenatal care
17. Childhood poverty
18. Proportion of persons living in counties exceeding Environmental Protection Agency (EPA) standards for air quality

*From Centers for Disease Control and Prevention, 1991.

sures that facilitate internal and external comparisons of an organization's performance over time (Loeb and Buck, 1996). One major performance indicator system is the Health Plan Employer Data and Information Set (HEDIS) (Corrigan and Nielsen, 1993). HEDIS was originally developed to compare the quality of care between and within managed care organizations (MCOs). For public health practitioners, an important aspect of HEDIS is its focus on issues that are amenable to primary and secondary prevention. For example, certain indicators in HEDIS (e.g., infant low birth weight and mammography screening) provide important tools for assessing program and intervention effectiveness within the MCO population.

Recently, the Institute of Medicine has discussed the use of performance indicators designed as important tools in the community health improvement process (Institute of Medicine, 1997). In addition, separate indicators for a community health profile were proposed to provide information on the community context in which health improvement efforts take place. The health profile indicators are grouped under six major headings: sociodemographic characteristics, health status, health risk factors, health care resource consumption, functional status, and quality of life. One of the goals of the set of proposed indicators is to bridge concepts of public health and health care in public and private settings.

Regardless of the potential usefulness of health indicators, the practical value of an indicator is dictated by the technical and organizational feasibility for collecting relevant data and the degree of precision required in the analysis. Re-

Table 8.6 Common Data Sources in Public Health Agencies that Provide Information Concerning Indicators

Vital events registries
Disease-specific registries
Population and house census
Routine health services records
Health programs delivery records
Hospital discharge data
Disease notification within surveillance systems
Sample surveys within surveillance systems
Other sample surveys
Other data banks from programs outside the health sector

sources in public health are always limited, and choosing an indicator that requires the establishment of a new surveillance system or intensive data collection may not be prudent. Recently, this trade-off has partly been alleviated as a result of the availability of computers, networking, and data consolidation strategies. New information technologies have allowed public health agencies access to several sources that collect information on health indicators that were previously unavailable (Table 8.6).

Indicators also can be organized according to the type of program evaluation being conducted (Table 8.7). Because outcome evaluation and indicators are covered in Chapter 9, the following discussion focuses on process and impact indicators. The distinctions between categories of indicators (e.g., process vs. impact) are not always distinct and have considerable overlap.

Process Indicators

Several factors should be considered in the process of program implementation, including (*1*) the characteristics of the population being served, (*2*) barriers to effective provision of health programs and services, (*3*) population expectations of the program, and (*4*) whether an adequate infrastructure exists to deliver the program (WHO, 1981b). To address these factors, indicators of process are usually measured against acceptable standards or norms for delivery of the program. In a typical public health project, indicators of process should encompass the following issues (Coyle et al., 1989) (Table 8.7):

- which target groups and subgroups are being served
- how persons learn about the services and what other services are available to them
- how a program learns about and reaches out to persons, engages them in receiving services, and limits attrition from the project

- what services and materials are delivered, by whom, how often, to whom, and in what context
- the accuracy and timeliness of the education or risk reduction information selected groups receive
- how resources are used

Impact Indicators

Because impact evaluation typically focuses on intermediate results occurring between program initiation and completion, impact indicators consist of measurable program/intervention outputs. The main question often is "Have the short-terms goals of a program been met?" In a typical health promotion program, an impact indicator focuses on the immediate impact of the intervention or program on one or more modifiable factors (e.g., knowledge, beliefs, attitudes, skills, social support, and behavior). Depending on the level of intervention, impact indicators can take differing forms (Table 8.8).

Often, health impact indicators form a subset of overall outcome indicators. For example, a consensus health status indicator in the United States is the breast cancer death rate (Table 8.5). The corresponding impact indicator might be the

Table 8.7 Indicators in Health Promotion and Education Programs*

Type	Health Indicator
Process, measures, program	Ratio of the number of instructors by group of recipients
	Percentage of learning activities completed by participants
	Ratio of the amount of resources budgeted by utilized (e.g., money, time, and personnel)
	Participants' satisfaction with health promotion education sessions
	Average time for health promotion and education
	Session by instructor
	Average number of participants per session
	Number of educational and information material distributed per session
Impact, measures, behavior	Percentage change in the prevalence of knowledge
	Percentage change in the prevalence of attitude
	Percentage change in the prevalence of habit
	Percentage change in score of skill
Outcome, measures, health outcomes	Mortality rate
	Incidence and/or discharge rate
	Disability rate - prevalence
	Prevalence of self-reported well-being

*Adapted from Green et al., 1980.

Table 8.8 Impact Evaluation Indicators According to the Level of Intervention*

Level of Intervention	Indicator
Individual	Mean score change of knowledge, belief, attitude among recipients
	Percentage change reduction in high-risk behavior in recipients
	Overall decrease of high-risk behavior in target population
Organizational	Adoption of a policy
	Percentage of programs personnel adopting policy
	Adoption of a program
	Size of resources allocated to program implementation
	Resources adequacy and appropriateness (budgeted/size of population)
Governmental	Adoption of legislation or regulation
	Number of actions taken to decrease opportunity for risk behavior
	Proportion of government budget allocated to program

*Adapted from Simons-Morton et al., 1995.

proportion of U.S. women aged 50 years or older who have undergone mammography and clinical breast exam within the past year.

Impact indicators for health care have been defined in a number of overlapping categories, including coverage, utilization, access, and quality. *Coverage* relates usage to the need within the health sector. It depends on the ability of the service to interact with those who need and should benefit from it. It is the proportion of the population who can receive or have received service (Morow, 1979; Vuori, 1982). *Utilization* is directly related to the number of persons who are in contact with the service. It is the relationship between the output and service capacity, which is generally expressed as a ratio of output given the capacity of the service. *Access* is defined as the number of persons who are potentially able to use the service. It is usually expressed as a proportion of the number of persons within a certain distance of the service in relation to the population in need of the service. Another challenging aspect of measuring health care relates to quality. A well-accepted definition of *quality* is its measurement through (*1*) structure (i.e., the characteristics of the resources of the health care system); (*2*) process (i.e., what is done to and for the patient); and (*3*) outcomes (i.e., the end results of the care process on the health and well-being of the patient) (Donabedian, 1988).

Statistical Issues

Numerous statistical and methodological issues are relevant to the topics of this chapter; some of these are covered in other chapters. Quasi-experimental designs were mentioned earlier in this chapter, and many of the statistical issues described relate to these designs (Koepsell et al., 1992).

Precision and Accuracy in Calculating Rates

Many of the processes of this chapter rely on the simple epidemiological tool—a rate. An incidence rate is the number of new cases of a disease per unit time per person-years at risk. Although the calculation of an incidence rate is not complex, important methodological issues underlie its development. If the numerator of the rate is dependent on a clinical diagnosis, bias in the definition of a case may influence the rate. Often, when implementing CQI or evaluating public health programs, sample sizes are small, making rates imprecise.

Sometimes, these calculations are called *small area analyses* because they are typically carried out at a subregional level. At this level, disease rates are unlikely to be routinely reported. As a rough guide, a "small area" has been defined as one containing fewer than 20 cases of the disease of interest (Cuzick and Elliott, 1992). Because small area analyses tend to deal with low-incidence events, special considerations and statistical tests may be necessary to deal with small numbers (Diehr et al., 1990).

Variability of Indicator Measures

An issue closely related to rate calculation is the estimation of the variability of an indicator in the planning, implementation, and evaluation of community-wide interventions. For example, one may need to know the variance around an estimate of dietary fat consumption in a community-wide study aimed at reducing serum cholesterol levels. Often, the "true" variability is underestimated. The common reason for this underestimation is that the variance of an indicator is often estimated at an individual level, whereas the intervention may be aimed at a community level. In other words, individuals are clustered within the sample allocated communities. The consequences of this error are usually reflected in an overestimate of statistical power and, hence, an underestimate of the sample size required to demonstrate the anticipated effect. Inappropriate statistical tests also may be used in the analyses that overestimate the intervention effects (Simpson et al., 1995).

Sample Size and Statistical Power

In the situations described in the previous section, two sources of variation have to be considered in both power calculation and data analysis: within-cluster variation (i.e., the mean squared deviation of individual responses within a cluster from the mean response for that cluster) and between-cluster variation (i.e., the mean squared deviation of the mean responses in the clusters from the overall mean). In addition, two types of sample size are considered—the number of persons per community and the number of communities per treatment [Koepsell (in press)]. For a cluster randomized trial involving c randomized communities to an intervention group and c more to a comparison group, with m persons studied per community, the variance of the mean for each intervention group is as follows:

$$\sigma_t^2 = \sigma_c^2/c + [(\sigma^2/m)/c] \qquad [8\text{--}1]$$

where σ_t, σ_c^2 and σ^2 are estimates of total variance, between and within cluster variances, respectively.

If the between-cluster variation is ignored, so that the total variance is the sum of the two components σ^2 and σ_c^2, the variability of the intervention effect is underestimated as

$$\sigma_t^2 = \sigma_c^2/mc + \sigma^2/mc \qquad [8\text{--}2]$$

and the sample size requirements will also be underestimated. The expression in Equation [8–1] also shows that as σ_c^2 gets large relative to σ^2 there is little gain from studying more persons per community (m), whereas including more communities in the study is likely to substantially increase study power. However, this strategy is limited when the number of clusters is small and expensive when the cluster size is large (Koepsell et al., 1992; Simpson et al., 1995). The limitation in the number of clusters is the main reason for a fixed number of persons studied; statistical power in classical analysis is almost always lower when allocation is by cluster rather than by individual (Cornfield, 1978). The small number of clusters and associated small numbers of degrees of freedom require higher critical values for test statistics than what would be needed had the sampling unit been the individual.

Because evaluators have no control over the size of either variances, they must rely on either one of two things to estimate an effective sample size: estimating both variances to perform correct power analysis or multiplying the sample size by a previously estimated *design effect* factor (D). Estimates of the community-level variance component for many risk factors, σ_c^2, can be made using available data sources [e.g., the Behavioral Risk Factor Surveillance System (BRFSS)] or previous studies. Using proposed statistical methods (Searle, 1987), some computer packages [e.g., the Statistical Analysis System (SAS) and Biomedical Programs (BMDP)], have procedures for variance component estimation. Both the SAS procedures (Proc Varcomp) and the BMDP (P3V) use maximum likelihood estimation (MLE) and restricted maximum likelihood estimation (RLME) methods in their estimation of variance component. Using a model approach and treating the clusters as random effects, the procedures estimate the variance of the random variable that is associated with the random effects (clusters); the "variance component" reveals how much of each of the random factors contribute to the overall variability in the dependent variable.

The design effect, or variance inflation factor (D), represents the amount by which the variance estimate obtained by ignoring cluster needs to be inflated to obtain the correct variance. It can also be theoretically defined as the ratio between estimate of variance under complex sample design by the variance originated from a simple random sample. It is usually estimated by:

$$D = 1 + (m-1)\,\rho$$

where ρ is the intraclass (or intracluster) correlation coefficient defined as $\rho = \sigma_c^2 / \sigma^2 + \sigma_c^2$, or the ratio of between-cluster variability to total variability.

Statistical Analysis

During analysis, estimates of the intervention (or factor) effect ignoring the clustering will lead to underestimation of standard errors and false narrowing of the confidence interval around estimates. In addition, the corresponding p-value would also be artificially low, leading to spuriously statistically significant intervention effect. Therefore, clustering must be taken into account in the analysis in two ways: (*1*) treating the cluster as the unit of analysis; and (*2*) treating the individual as the unit of analysis, but taking ρ into account.

The first approach would make the aggregated summary statistic for all persons in each cluster the outcome variable (e.g., mean change in dietary fat intake). The intervention effect would then be estimated using the bivariate or multivariate method. When using multivariate techniques, adjustment to covariates would only be possible at the cluster level (e.g., cluster size, location, index of poverty). Also, this approach is limited to applications with balanced designs (i.e., same size per group or block).

In the second approach, the individual is the unit of analysis, and the correlation between responses of persons in the same cluster should be addressed through appropriate methods (Donner and Klar, 1994; Graubard and Korn, 1994). Some of these techniques include mixed-effect models analysis of variance (or covariance) with cluster nested within treatment groups for a continuous dependent variable; generalized estimating equations; and other techniques. These regression techniques are fully described elsewhere for categorical dependent variables (Graubard and Korn, 1994; Zeger et al., 1988). From a practical standpoint, major statistical software packages (e.g., SAS and BMDP) have the ability to conduct these analyses. However, the researcher/evaluator should be aware of assumptions about the statistical properties of test statistics generated. Occasionally, it is better for a researcher/evaluator to specify the model desired using random, fixed, and mixed effects with nesting within clusters, rather than using available contrasts in the package procedures. This will prevent spurious statistically significant results.

Improving Validity and Reliability

An important related issue involves the validity and reliability of measurement instruments (see also Chapter 9). *Reliability* is the extent to which results of a measurement can be replicated, and validity is the extent to which an instrument measures what it purports to measure [Petitti et al. (1991)]. *Validity* can be further subdivided into two questions: (*1*) Can the observed results be attributed to the program or intervention (i.e., internal validity)? and (*2*) Can the observed results be generalized to other settings or subjects (i.e., external validity)? Health care researchers need valid and reliable information on the effectiveness, efficiency, and methods for delivering health care and promoting healthy lifestyle, which can only be obtained through the use of scientifically sound evaluation research (Fink, 1992).

Despite the widespread use of CQI methods, relatively few systematic evaluations have been conducted on the effectiveness of CQI, and the development of valid and reliable measurement tools for CQI is limited. The relationships among organizational culture, quality improvement processes, and selected outcomes in a sample of 61 U.S. hospitals have recently been studied (Shortell et al., 1995b). There were several important aspects of this study. First, a conceptual model was developed a priori, with specific hypotheses related to model constructs. Second, tested scales and questionnaires were used in the study and a statistical measure (Cronbach's α) was used to test the reliability of the scales. Third, established performance indicators were used to measure organizational characteristics relevant to the study.

In addition to being valid and reliable, measurement tools and indicators need to be *sensitive* to the changes in the situation they are supposed to measure, *specific* to reflect changes only in the situation concerned, and *objective* to provide the same answer if measured by different persons. A few recommendations may be useful to public health professionals as they attempt to implement more valid and reliable interventions:

- Pilot testing before conducting a full study can help to identify evidence of concordance and discordance in various evaluation measures.
- External validity is more likely when indicators are generated from random samples of the target population. If possible, it is useful to stratify and randomly select a sample from within each heterogeneous group of persons, places, or times.

- Development of a program theory (e.g., a "causal model") can lead to selection of appropriate process and impact indicators. A range of program staff and policymakers should generally be involved in model development. Frameworks for these models are available in the literature (e.g., Goodman and Wandersman, 1994).

Measuring Temporal Trends in Public Health Indicators

Often, data on public health indicators are collected over a period of time (e.g., months or years). To determine whether public health programs are effective, *trend analyses* frequently must be conducted. Trend analyses of selected indicators seek to answer the questions: "How much has been accomplished?" and "How fast are program objectives being met?" A recent example of a time-series analysis is a study of the decrease in firearm fatalities in Washington, DC, following implementation of gun control legislation (Loftin et al., 1991). Data led researchers to conclude that restrictive licensing of handguns was associated with a prompt decline in homicides and suicides by firearms.

Many statistical techniques can be used to track progress or make predictions based on indicators—for example, linear regression, time-series analysis, plotting of moving averages, log-linear modeling, and Poisson regression.

In some cases, a simple linear regression model will fit the data. A more complicated method for time-series analysis is auto regressive integrated moving average (ARIMA) modeling (Box and Jenkins, 1976). ARIMA models are for relatively long series of data and have an advantage over other modeling methods in that they account for period-to-period correlations (Stroup, 1994). Recently, Poisson regression has been used as a prediction model for incidence rates. The Poisson distribution is a distribution function designed to test the occurrence of rare events in a continuum of time or space (Last, 1995). The number of events has a Poisson distribution with parameter λ (lambda) if the probability of observing k events ($k = 0, 1, \ldots$) is equal to:

$$p(x = k) = (e^{-\lambda} \lambda^k) / k!$$

where e is the base of natural logarithm (2.7183), the mean and variance of the distribution are both equal to λ.

Predicting Cross-Sectional Associations

In most public health practice settings, extensive etiological research (e.g., case-control studies or prospective cohort studies) is not conducted. However, in many public health settings, an array of cross-sectional data are available to study cross-sectional associations. Although these associations cannot be considered causal, they can be valuable in program planning efforts.

The statistical method of logistic regression can be useful in studying "predictors" of a health behavior. The logistic regression model is a model for probability. It models the probability of an event occurrence, a risk for an individual of having the outcome of interest, conditional on a vector of independent (explanatory) variables. In a typical epidemiological context, assume a researcher observed independent variables, $X_1, X_2, X_3, \ldots X_i$, in a group of subjects for whom outcome status is determined as 1 if "with outcome" and 0 if "without the outcome." This information is used to describe the probability that the outcome will occur (risk) during a defined period of time (T_0 to T_1) as follows:

$$P(D = 1 \mid X_1, X_2, X_3, \ldots X_i)$$
$$= 1 / 1 + \exp - (\alpha + \sum \beta_i X_i)$$

In this epidemiological context (following subjects from time T_0 to T_1 to measure occurrence of event), the ratio of the risk of a subject with certain characteristics ($X_1 = 1$) by another subject without the characteristic ($X_1 = 0$) is then referred as the relative risk, or risk ratio. In addition, the ratio of the odds $[p(D = 1|X)]/1 - [P(D = 1|X)]$ of subjects with the characteristic ($X = 1$) to the odds of subjects without the characteristic ($X = 0$) can be used to generate the risk odds ratio (ROR).

The odds ratio based on the logistic model can also be expressed as:

$$\ln \text{ odds ratio} = \ln \{[p(D = 1|X)]/1 - [P(D = 1|X)]\} = \alpha + \sum \beta_i X_i$$

The β represents the change in ln odds that would result from one unit change in the variable X_1 when all other X's are fixed.

To illustrate how a state health department can use cross-sectional data to examine population-based health issues, a study from Missouri is briefly described [Hagdrup et al. (in press)]. Researchers used logistic regression and the BRFSS (Remington, et al. 1988; Gentry, et al. 1985) to examine health care coverage in relation to various predictors of health care coverage. "Preventive" health care coverage was defined as self-reported availability of a health plan and coverage for all or most preventive services. After adjusting for sociodemographic and behavioral risk factors with logistic regression, persons age younger than 65 years were almost one-third as likely to have full preventive coverage compared with persons aged 65 years or older.

Use of Generalized Linear Models

Another group of regression techniques useful in evaluating impact of public health programs is generalized linear models. This class of regression models is an extension of linear regression in which the dependent variable is continuous and the independent variables are a combination of nominal and interval variables. It includes multivariate linear models, analysis of covariance, and analysis of variance. Effects can enter models as fixed, random, and mixed. The fixed effect is present when the levels of the factors are unique. When the levels of a factor are a set (sample) of many other possible levels, it is defined as random effect. A mixed-effect model would include both fixed and random effects in the model.

Researchers used generalized linear models to identify sociodemographic and health-related behaviors associated with dietary fat intake from a large population-based cross-sectional survey including most U.S. states (Simoes et al., 1995).

Survival Analysis

In survival analysis, the interest is in determining the probability of an event occurrence in relation to the amount of time until its occurrence for each subject in the study. The outcome of interest is, therefore, the time until event occurrence. The event usually is defined as a failure (e.g., death, recidivism, or relapse) and is coded as a binary variable. For program evaluation, the time between exposure to program intervention and the event occurrence is the critical information for computing the survival function. The concept of censoring and how it is used in the analysis is critical to the understanding of survival analysis and related methods. Censoring occurs when the investigator has some information about individual survival time but does not know the exact survival time; thus, the investigator can only ensure that a subject survived up to a certain time or longer. Only two possibilities exist: a subject either failed or was censored.

Survival models can also be useful in the evaluation of immediate outputs of health programs. For example, in a human immunodeficiency virus (HIV) health education and counseling program, the major objective is to keep risky behavior at a minimum so that subjects and contacts minimize their chances of getting infected with and transmitting HIV. In this situation, HIV-identified persons are counseled and followed-up for assessment of their risk behavior over time. If their behavior shows no improvement after subsequent health education and counseling sessions, more aggressive measures may be taken. The effects of counseling and education can be evaluated using survival models. The outcome of interest is the failure to change behavior or recidivism of high-risk behavior (e.g., needle sharing and unprotected sex). Because subjects are followed-up, their survival time (i.e., the time with improved behavior) can be measured. The effect of intervention on high-risk behavior could be evaluated controlling for other factors.

Case Study: "Give Me 5" School-Based Program to Increase Fruit and Vegetable Consumption

Background

Epidemiological studies have shown that higher consumption of fruits and vegetables is associated with decreased risk of several chronic diseases (e.g., colon cancer and coronary heart disease) (Negri et al., 1991; Gaziano et al., 1992). Because childhood eating habits can predict fruit and vegetable intake as an adult (Krebs-Smith et al., 1995), establishing healthy eating practices early in life is an important public health intervention.

Modeled after the "5 A Day—For Better Health" project conducted in California that focused largely on adults (Foerster and Bal, 1990), the "Give Me 5" program is designed to increase fruit and vegetable consumption among elementary school students. The Missouri Department of Health is currently implementing and evaluating the Give Me 5 program. Materials were modified from those being used in Massachusetts.

The overall goal of Give Me 5 is to establish lifelong healthy eating habits among second grade students. The two objectives of the program are to (*1*) increase the number of participating schools to 100% by the year 2000 and (*2*) increase fruit and vegetable consumption among the target population. The basis of the program is a curriculum book with eight activities designed to familiarize students with a wide variety of fruits and vegetables and the benefits of healthy eating. Students are encouraged to pledge to eat five or more servings of fruits and vegetables per day.

Study Design

A quasi-experimental design is being used to evaluate the effectiveness of the Give Me 5 program. Classrooms were divided into intervention and comparison groups. Intervention classrooms ($n = 60$) receive the Give Me 5 activities and evaluation; comparison classrooms ($n = 60$) will not receive the intervention but will be evaluated. Evaluation data will derive from four primary sources: (*1*) administrative data from participating teachers; (*2*) a sample of the fruit and vegetable content of menus from intervention and comparison schools; (*3*) a two-question food-frequency survey of children; and (*4*) a brief survey of parents/guardians on the children's eating habits.

Discussion Issues

Several process indicators can be measured primarily with administrative data, including: (*1*) the number of teachers participating, (*2*) the number of students participating, (*3*) the number of Give Me 5 activities conducted in each classroom over time, (*4*) the amount of time devoted to the program in each classroom, (*5*) the satisfaction of teachers with the program, and (*6*) the cost of the program per student. Impact indicators will derive primarily from the food frequency questionnaires. The primary impact indicator is the percentage change in consumption of fruit and vegetable intake in intervention children versus comparison children.

Sample size calculations are based on the method described by Simpson et al. (1995). As discussed previously, an estimate of the intraclass correlation coefficient is necessary to estimate how much the sample size needs to be inflated. Because no reliable data are currently available on fruit and vegetable consumption among Missouri children, the Missouri Behavioral Risk Factor Surveillance System was used to estimate the prevalence and intraclass correlation. Based on these estimates and assuming a 50% response rate on the food frequency questionnaire, a sample of 60 classrooms will result in approximately 600 students in intervention and comparison groups. This sample will detect a difference of 10% between intervention and comparison groups in fruit and vegetable consumption.

CQI and Application of Results

Although this project does not formally use CQI methods, several pieces of the CQI model are present in the design and implementation of the project. For example, in the design of Give Me 5, the "customers" (i.e., children) were involved in development of the evaluation instruments. In addition, the extensive process evaluation built into the project will provide feedback loops that should help with midcourse corrections in the program.

Results of the program will be disseminated among multiple audiences, including (*1*) students, teachers, and parents/guardians participating the study; (*2*) public health practitioners and academic researchers via presentations and publication of findings in a peer-reviewed journal; (*3*) other managers and decision makers in the health department; and (*4*) if effective, policymakers in the governor's office and state legislature to obtain resources for replication.

Strengths and Limitations

Many programs in the public health setting are implemented and continued without sufficient evaluation and monitoring. This study will provide scientifically sound information on a public health program that can be used in future program planning. The study operates on a small budget, and therefore, evaluation approaches are limited. For example, program staff are anticipating a 50% response rate from students on the food frequency questionnaire. This rate is lower than optimal in a rigorous research study. Applied research in the public health setting must balance what is scientifically rigorous with what is programmatically feasible.

Areas for Future Development

Applying and Evaluating CQI in the Public Health Setting

As noted earlier, only limited research has been conducted on the uses and effectiveness of CQI methods in the public health setting. Although CQI originally was developed to improve efficiency in manufacturing and business, many aspects of a CQI model have appeal and relevance to public health practice.

Measuring the Effects of Indicator Use on Public Health Practice

Increasingly, public health agencies report on indicators that are being used to track progress (e.g., Sutocky et al., 1996). However, limited research exists regarding whether systematic use of indicators improves program delivery and effectiveness.

Implementing and Evaluating New Training Programs

Persons often enter the field of public health practice from a variety of educational backgrounds, frequently lacking formal training in a public health discipline (e.g., epidemiology or biostatistics). Therefore, a need exists for "on-the-job" training programs in public health agencies. Presently, few such training programs exist with a significant focus on use of quantitative methods to improve program implementation, management, and evaluation. These training programs are needed, especially those with strong components to evaluate their effectiveness.

Practice–Academic Linkages

Each of the preceding issues can benefit from close interactions between public health agencies and academic institutions (e.g., schools of public health, departments of preventive medicine) [Brownson and Kreuter (in press)]. In certain cases, practice–academic collaborations have led to new teaching opportunities in management and leadership (Capper et al., 1996). The CDC's "Centers for Research and Demonstration of Health Promotion and Disease Prevention" also demonstrate beneficial linkages between public health agencies and academic institutions (Institute of Medicine, 1997).

Public Health–Health Care Linkages

Primarily due to concern about rising costs, the U.S. health care system currently is undergoing profound changes that will influence the practice of public health in the coming decade. Health maintenance organizations have grown from enrollments of 6 million persons in 1976 to 46 million in 1995 (National Center for Health Statistics, 1996b). Within the next decade, 80%–90% of the insured U.S. population will receive its health care through various forms of managed care (Pew Health Professions Commission, 1995). There are many opportunities for collaborations between public health and health care in implementing and evaluating new health programs.

Conclusion

A wide array of programmatic and statistical tools are available to the public health manager. Although little research has been conducted on the effectiveness of the use of quantitative methods to manage and implement public health programs, the use of these methods likely will improve public health practice.

References

Anonymous. The quality march. National survey profiles quality improvement activities. *Hosp. Health Netw.* 67:52, 54–55, 1993.

Arrington, B., K. Gautam, and W. J. McCabe. Continually improving governance. *Hosp. Health Serv. Admin.* 40:95–110, 1995.

Berwick, D. M., A. B. Godfrey, and J. Roessner. *Curing Health Care. New Strategies for Quality Improvement.* San Francisco, CA: Jossey-Bass Publishers, 1991.

Box, G. E. P., and G. M. Jenkins. Some statistical aspects of adaptive optimization and control. *J. R. Stat. Soc.* 24:297–343, 1962.

Box, G. E. P., and G. Jenkins. *Time Series Analysis: Forecasting Control.* San Francisco, CA: Holden-Day, 1976.

Breslow, L. The future of public health: prospects in the United States for the 1990s. *Annu. Rev. Public Health* 11:1–28, 1990.

Brownson, R. C., and M. W. Kreuter. Future trends affecting public health: challenges and opportunities. *J. Public Health Manage. Pract.* 3:49–60, 1997.

Capper, S. A., W. J. Duncan, P. M. Ginter, C. Barganier, N. Blough, and P. Cleaveland. Translating public health research into public health practice: outcomes and characteristics of successful collaborations. *Am. J. Prev. Med.* 12(Suppl. 1):S67–S70, 1996.

Centers for Disease Control and Prevention. Consensus set of health status indicators for the general assessment of community health status—United States. *MMWR Morb. Mortal. Wkly. Rep.* 40:449–451, 1991.

Centers for Disease Control and Prevention. *Planned Approach to Community Health (PATCH): Program Description.* Atlanta, GA: U.S. Public Health Service, Centers for Disease Control, 1992.

Centers for Disease Control and Prevention. *CDC's Tobacco Use Prevention Program: Working Toward a Healthier Future. At-A-Glance.* Atlanta, GA: Centers for Disease Control and Prevention, 1996.

Cornfield, J. Randomization by group: a formal analysis. *Am. J. Epidemiol.* 108:100–102, 1978.

Corrigan, J. M., and D. M. Nielsen. Toward the development of uniform reporting standards for managed care organizations: the Health Plan Employer Data and Information Set (Version 2.0). *Jt. Comm. J. Qual. Improv.* 19:566–575, 1993.

Coyle, S. L., R. F. Boruch, and C. F. Turner, (Eds.). *Evaluating AIDS Prevention Programs.* Washington, DC: National Research Council, National Academy Press, 1989.

Cuzick, J., and P. Elliott. Small area studies: purpose and methods. In: *Geographical and Environmental Epidemiology: Methods for Small Area Studies,* edited by P. Elliot, J. Cuzick, D. English, and R. Stern. Oxford: Oxford University Press, 1992, pp. 14–21.

Deming, W. E. *Sample Design in Business Research.* New York: John Wiley & Sons, 1960.

Deming, W. E. *Out of the Crisis.* Cambridge, MA: MIT-CAES, 1986.

Diehr, P., K. Cain, F. Connell, and E. Volinn. What is too much variation? The null hypothesis in small-area analysis. *Health Serv. Res.* 24:741–771, 1990.

Donabedian, A. The quality of care: how can it be assessed? *JAMA* 260:1743–1748, 1988.

Donner, A., and N. Klar. Methods for comparing event rates in intervention studies when the unit of allocation is a cluster. *Am. J. Epidemiol.* 140:279–289, 1994.

Dyal, W. W. *Public Health Infrastructure and Organizational Practices Definitions.* Atlanta, GA: Public Health Practice Program Office, Centers for Disease Control, DHHS, August 22, 1991.

Dyal, W. W. Ten organizational practices of public health: a historical perspective. *Am. J. Prev. Med.* 11(Suppl. 2):S6–S8, 1995.

Ferris, L. E., and J. I. Williams. Authors' response. *Can. Med. Assoc. J.* 147:1117–1118, 1992.

Fink, A. A program evaluation in health care. *Can. Med. Assn. J.* 147:1116–1118, 1992.

Foerster, S. B., and D. G. Bal. California's "5 A Day—For Better Health" campaign. *Chronic Dis. Notes Rep.* 3:7–9, 1990.

Gaziano, J. M., J. E. Manson, J. E. Buring, and C. H. Hennekens. Dietary antioxidants and cardiovascular diseases. *Ann. N. Y. Acad. Sci.* 669:249–259, 1992.

Gentry, E. M., W. D. Kalsbeek, G. C. Hogelin, et al. The behavioral risk factor surveys: design, methods, and estimates from combined state data. *Am. J. Prev. Med.* 1:9–14, 1985.

Goodman, R. M., and A. Wandersman. FORECAST: a formative approach to evaluating community coalitions and community-based interventions. In: Monograph Series CSAP Special Issue, edited by S. J. Kartarian, and W. B. Hansen. *J. Commun. Psych.* 1994, pp. 6–25.

Graubard, B. I., and E. L. Korn. Regression analysis with clustered data [Review]. *Stat. Med.* 13:509–522, 1994.

Green, L. W., and M. W. Kreuter. *Health Promotion Planning: An Educational and Environmental Approach,* 2nd ed. Mountain View, CA: Mayfield, 1991.

Green, L. W., and F. M. Lewis. *Measurement and Evaluation in Health Education and Health Promotion.* Palo Alto, CA: Mayfield, 1986.

Haddock, CC, C. Nosky, C. A. Fargason, and R. S. Kurz. The impact of CQI on human resources management. *Hosp. Health Serv. Admin.* 40:138–153, 1995.

Hagdrup, N., E. J. Simoes, and R. C. Brownson. Health care coverage: traditional and preventive measures and associations with chronic disease risk factors. *J. Community Health* 22:387–399, 1997.

Hamaker, H. C., E. S. Page, and M. Zelen. Quality control, statistical. In: *International Encyclopedia of Statistics,* edited by W. H. Kruskal, and J. M. Tanur. New York: Macmillan, 1978, pp. 803–812.

Holland, W.W. *Measurements in Health Care.* New York: Oxford University Press, 1983.

Institute of Medicine, Committee for the Study of the Future of Public Health, Institute of Medicine. *The Future of Public Health.* Washington, DC: National Academy Press, 1988.

Institute of Medicine. *Linking Research and Public Health Practice: Review of CDC's program of Centers for Research and Demonstration of Health Promotion and Disease Prevention.* Washington, DC: Institute of Medicine, National Academy Press, 1997.

Kaluzny, A. D., C. P. McLaughlin, and K. Simpson. Applying total quality management concepts to public health organizations. *Public Health Rep.* 107:257–264, 1992.

Kaluzny, A. D., C. P. McLaughlin, and D. Kibbe. Quality improvement: beyond the institution. *Hosp. Health Serv. Admin.* 40:172–188, 1995.

Koepsell, T. D., E. H. Wagner, and A. C. Cheadle. Selected methodological issues in evaluating community-based health promotion and disease prevention issues. *Annu. Rev. Public Health* 13:31–57, 1992.

Koepsell, T. Epidemiologic issues in the evaluation of community intervention trials. In: *Applied Epidemiology: Theory to Practice,* edited by R. C. Brownson, and D. B. Petitti. New York: Oxford University Press, 1998.

Krebs-Smith, S. M., J. Keimendinger, B. H. Patterson, A. F. Subar, R. Kessler, and E. Pivonka. Psychosocial factors associated with fruit and vegetable consumption. *J. Health Promo.* 10:98–104, 1995.

Last, J. M. (ed.). *A Dictionary of Epidemiology,* 3rd ed. New York: Oxford University Press, 1995.

Loeb, J. M., and A. S. Buck. From the Joint Commission on the Accreditation of Healthcare Organizations. *JAMA* 275(7):508, 1996.

Loftin, C., D. McDowall, B. Wiersema, and T. J. Cottey. Effects of restrictive licensing of handguns on homicide and suicide in the District of Columbia. *N. Engl. J. Med.* 325:1615–1620, 1991.

McLaughlin, C. P., and A. D. Kaluzny. *Continuous Improvement in Health Care: Theory, Implementation and Applications.* Gaithersburg, MD: Aspen Publishers, 1994.

Miller, C. A., K. S. Moore, T. B. Richards, and J. D. Monk. A proposed method for assessing the performance of local public health functions and practices. *Am. J. Public Health* 84:1743–1749, 1994.

Morow, R. H. Measurements of coverage, effectiveness, and efficiency of health care in less developed countries. Draft background paper prepared for WHO workshop, January 1979.

National Association of County Health Officials. *Assessment Protocol for Excellence in Public Health (APEX-PH).* Washington, DC: NACHO, 1991.

National Association of County and City Health Officials. *1992–1993 national profile of local health departments. National Surveillance Series.* Washington, DC: National Association of County and City Health Officials, 1995.

National Center for Health Statistics. *Healthy People 2000 Review, 1995–96.* Hyattsville,

MD: U.S. Department of Health and Human Services, Public Health Service, DHHS Publication No. (PHS)96–1256, 1996a.

National Center for Health Statistics. *Health, United States, 1995.* Hyattsville, MD: U.S. Department of Health and Human Services, Public Health Service, DHHS Publication No. (PHS)96–1232, 1996b.

Negri, E., C. La Vecchia, S. Franceschi, B. D'Avanzo, and F. Parazzini. Vegetable and fruit consumption and cancer risk. *Int. J. Cancer* 48:350–354, 1991.

Oberle, M. W., E. L. Baker, and M. J. Magenheim. Healthy people 2000 and community health planning. *Annu. Rev. Public Health* 15:259–275, 1994.

Osborne, D., and T. Gaebler. *Reinventing Government: How the Entrepreneurial Spirit is Transforming the Public Sector.* New York: Penguin Books USA Inc., 1992.

Petitti, D. B., R. C. Brownson, and A. C. King. Epidemiologic methods and applications. In: *Applied Epidemiology: Theory to Practice,* edited by R. C. Brownson, and D. B. Petitti. New York: Oxford University Press, 1991.

Pew Health Professions Commission. *Critical Challenges: Revitalizing the Health Professions for the Twenty-First Century.* The Third Report of the Pew Health Commission. San Francisco, CA: UCSF Center for the Health Professions, 1995.

Remington, P. L., M. Y. Smith, D. F. Williamson, R. F. Anda, E. M. Gentry, and G. C. Hogelin. Design, characteristics, and usefulness of state-based behavioral risk factor surveillance: 1981–87. *Public Health Rep.* 103:366–375, 1988.

Searle, S. R. *Linear Models for Unbalanced Data.* New York: John Wiley & Sons, 1987.

Shortell, S. M., D. Z. Levin, J. L. O'Brien, and H.F.X. Hughes. Assessing the evidence on CQI: is the glass half empty or half full? *Hosp. Health Serv. Admin.* 40:4–24, 1995a.

Shortell, S. M., J. L. O'Brien, J. M. Carman, et al. Assessing the impact of continuous quality improvement/total quality management: concept versus implementation. *Health Serv. Res.* 30:377–401, 1995b.

Siegfried, J. Largest tobacco-control program begins. *J. Natl. Cancer Inst.* 83:1446–1447, 1991.

Simoes, E. J., T. Byers, R. J. Coates, M. K. Serdula, A. H. Mokdad, and G. W. Heath. The association between leisure-time physical activity and dietary fat in American adults. *Am. J. Public Health* 85:240–244, 1995.

Simons-Morton, B. G, W. H. Greene, and N. H. Gottlieb. *Introduction to Health Education and Health Promotion,* 2nd ed. Prospect Heights, IL: Waveland Press, Inc., 1995.

Simons-Morton, D. G., B. G. Simons-Morton, G. S. Parcel, and J. F. Bunker. Influencing personal and environmental conditions for community health: a multilevel intervention model. *Fam. Community Health* 11:25–35, 1988.

Simpson, J. M., N. Klar, and A. Donner. Accounting for cluster randomization: a review of primary prevention trials, 1990 through 1993. *Am. J. Public Health* 85:1378–1383, 1995.

Stroup, D. F. Special analytic issues. In: *Principles and Practices of Public Health Surveillance,* edited by S. M. Teutsch, and R. E. Churchill. New York: Oxford University Press, 1994, pp. 136–149.

Sutocky, J. W., S. Dumbauld, and G. B. Abbott. Year 2000 health status indicators: a profile of California. *Public Health Rep.* 111:521–526, 1996.

Turnock, B. J., A. Handler, W. W. Dyal, et al. Implementing and assessing organizational practices in local health departments. *Public Health Rep.* 109:478–484, 1994.

U.S. Public Health Service. *Healthy People 2000: National Health Promotion and Disease Prevention.* Washington, DC: U.S. Department of Health and Human Services, Public Health Service, DHHS Publication No. 017–001–00473–1, 1990.

Vuori, H. V. *Quality Assurance of Health Services: Concepts and Methods.* Copenhagen: World Health Organization, 1982.

World Health Organization. *Health Program Evaluation: Guiding Principles for its Application in the Managerial Process for National Development.* Health for All Series, No. 6 Geneva: World Health Organization, 1981a.

World Health Organization. *Managerial Process from National Health Development. Guiding Principles for Use and Support for Health For All by Year 2000.* Health for All Series No. 5. Geneva: World Health Organization, 1981b.

Zeger, S. L., K. Y. Liang, and P. S. Albert. Models for longitudinal data: a generalized estimating equation approach. *Biometrics* 44:1049–1060, 1988.

Zucconi, S. L., and C. A. Carson. CDC's consensus set of health status indicators: monitoring and prioritization by state health departments. *Am. J. Public Health* 84: 1644–1646, 1994.

9

Evaluation

MICHAEL HENNESSY

> The techniqes that evaluators may bring to bear are only tools, and
> even the very best of tools do not ensure a worthy product. Just as
> for any craft, there is no substitute for intelligence, experience, per-
> severence, and a touch of whimsy.
>
> —Richard Berk and Peter Rossi

In 1987, federal regulations limited the application of physical restraint methods in nursing homes in the United States. Did these regulations actually reduce the use of restraints? What is the best way to retrain staff of nursing homes to comply with these regulations? (Phillips et al., 1993; Dunbar et al., 1996).

By 1995, 506,538 cases of acquired immunodeficiency syndrome (AIDS) among adults and adolescents in the United States were reported to the Centers for Disease Control and Prevention (CDC). What approach to counseling and testing for human immunodeficiency virus (HIV) is the most effective in preventing the spread of HIV infection? (U.S. Preventive Services Task Force, 1996).

Among public health measures to reduce alcohol-related motor vehicle fatalities and injuries are responsible beverage service practices and policies in commercial establishments, local and state regulations restricting alcohol sales and availability, media campaigns targeted at drinking and driving, and technological changes in automobiles and roads that reduce the risk of drinking and driving. Which combination of these alternative programs will maximally reduce morbid ity and mortality on the highways? (Delewski and Saltz, 1990; Casswell et al., 1989; Ross, 1992; Holder et al., 1997).

The management of diabetes mellitus depends on modifying behavioral risks and learning a repertoire of appropriate care management techniques and skills. What are the barriers to preventive self-care in this population? (Graham, 1991; Hampson et al., 1995).

Each of these questions involves policy, procedural, health promotion, or clinical changes in standard public health practices. Each question also addresses the relative superiority or the changing temporal effects of actual or potential alterations in the status quo. Thus, the questions define the essential problem of *program evaluation,* which involves scientific methods for planning, implementing, and assessing the effects of policies and interventions. Given the range of public health issues and the diversity and values of parties interested in the outcomes of evaluations, answering questions such as those posed above is often politically sensitive and scientifically complicated.

The evaluation process is political because different policy options usually reflect the values of influential groups such as owners and employees of nursing homes, AIDS activists, Mothers Against Drunk Drivers (MADD), and proponents of media advocacy (Wallack and Dorfman, 1996). Interested parties may have preconceived notions of how they will use evaluation results such as advocating for program maintenance or program termination regardless of program effectiveness (Dial, 1994; Worthen, 1995; Hennessy and Sullivan, 1989).

Evaluation of public health programs is also complicated scientifically by the fact that it is often carried out under conditions of low experimental control, in contrast to the usual practices in the biological and physical sciences. Thus, careful attention to the design of evaluations is important to appropriate causal inferences. Evaluators attempt to compensate for inadequate experimental control in several ways, but the problem remains universal.

Effective Evaluation

For most purposes, a complete evaluation includes at least the following three interrelated elements and should be carried out sequentially (Short et al., 1996):

- program design and development
- program monitoring tasks
- program impact estimation

Evaluators have much to contribute to the design of programs (Kennedy, 1983; Fitzpatrick, 1988; McClintock, 1990; Dumka et al., 1995). However, program design is one of the most difficult tasks because the questions raised concerning design are fundamental and usually have theoretical and administrative (but not technical) answers (Smith, 1989). For example, while all parties must agree on the goals of the program, the need to define the program goals may reveal conflicts among stakeholders that require resolution (e.g., Kaskutas et al., 1991–92). Clarification of the goals should enhance program design and operation and facilitate meaningful evaluation (Pentz et al., 1996).

Program monitoring (often called process evaluation) should document actual program functioning (Dehar et al., 1993; Finnegan et al., 1989), measure exposure to and diffusion of the intervention treatments (Fortmann et al., 1982; Hausman et al., 1992; Steckler et al., 1992), and identify barriers to implementation (Demers and Renaud, 1992). This component asks which elements of the program were actually implemented. The evaluation plan should ensure that data are readily available to answer the question, because perspectives on which elements were actually carried out may differ among stakeholders in the absence of documentation.

Empirically documenting program functioning is important for two reasons. First, if the program is a success, other persons will be interested in replicating the results in other locations that serve other populations. Second, if the program is a failure, understanding exactly how each component of the program did or did not work is imperative (Chen, 1990). Treating social programs as a black box problem with no knowledge of the mechanisms within is a mistake (Lipsey, 1993; Short and Hennessy, 1994). In addition, knowledge of the adaptation of programs to their environments may provide important clues about how the programs actually operate and facilitate improvement.

Finally, outcome analysis looks at the effectiveness of the actual program. Such analysis includes two tasks: (1) defining program impact and (2) designing the impact study. Defining program impact includes identifying measurable outcomes. Identifying such outcomes is often difficult because the evaluator must link the theoretical goals of the program (as defined in the program design stage) to empirical and measurable indicators in the "real world." For example, reviews of measurement problems concerning sexually transmitted disease (STD), HIV, long-term care, and alcohol use can be found in Aral and Peterman (1996), Leviton and Valdiserri (1990), Hennessy and Hennessy (1990), and Saltz et al. (1992), respectively.

The impact evaluation must be designed to ensure a change recorded in the measurements is caused by the actions of the program and not by other external or internal influences. External influences are always a potential explanation for program outcome. In an evaluation of the effects of drug abuse prevention programs (Hansen, 1992), positive results of a school intervention might be caused by a change in the local availability of illicit drugs and not program effectiveness. Internal influences also need to be considered. For example, instructional programs that use computers to train medical students (Brown and Carlson, 1990) may purposively (e.g., through selectively enrolling those with prior computer experience) or inadvertently (e.g., through respondent volunteering) select persons to participate who are already computer literate. Any gains discovered probably represent an unrealistically high estimate of program efficacy compared with results obtained from participants who have no preexisting computer skills.

Performing Evaluations

The components of a scientifically valid evaluation are generally accepted (e.g., Green and Lewis, 1986; Rossi and Freeman, 1993, Windsor et al., 1994). However, evaluations may be conducted differently for different audiences. For example, some evaluations use a program's stated goals and outcomes to define the research problem, whereas other studies explicitly ignore the program's goals and objectives (Scriven, 1994). Evaluations may be intended for policy and decision makers and/or program administrators (Berk and Rossi, 1990) or for program clients (Fetterman, 1994). Evaluation may be seen as a cooperative enterprise in the construction of a shared "meaning" of a program that is essentially qualitative to better assess its worth between groups of stakeholders (Guba and Lincoln, 1989). Evaluation processes may also reflect a tradition of half a century of clinical and/or educational randomized experiments that are essentially quantitative (Campbell and Stanley, 1966). In addition, on an operational level, the usefulness of evaluation results may manifest themselves in programmatic improvements (Cronbach, 1982).

Methodology of Evaluation

Multiple methodologies have evolved from the scientific disciplines that have been used to answer the diversity of evaluation questions (Patton, 1996). While no single method is common to all evaluations or used by all evaluators, four criteria often are applied to specific instances to assess the quality of a particular evaluation. These common criteria are re-statements of the four "types of validity" developed by Cook and Campbell (1979):

Statistical conclusion validity: Does the evaluation design allow for accurate measures of relationships between variables and the presence of sampling error?

Construct validity: Does the evaluation design allow for valid measures and scales?

Internal validity: Does the evaluation design allow for causal attribution of relationships between variables?

External validity: Does the evaluation design provide generalizable results across other times, locations, and subjects?

Although this terminology may connote other concepts used in social research, the terms are widely accepted in evaluation and other social sciences. Evaluation designs that address each of the four questions posed by the type of validity yield research plans with the following characteristics:

- unambiguous relationships between variables (i.e., the likelihood of sampling error alone producing the observed associations is minimal)
- clear meaning between the theoretical concepts and the observed measures
- lack of alternative causal explanations for the observed relationships
- appropriately representative samples of subjects, locations, and times

In this chapter, the four types of validity are discussed in detail because they pose particular statistical challenges to the evaluation. However, before the statistical implications of these four types of validity are discussed, notice that the optimal combination of these types and each of the four types of validity alone do not indicate any preference about a particular research method or a particular evaluation problem. Rather, they refer to the evaluation plan, which includes elements pertaining to statistical inference, the quality of empirical measures, the legitimacy of causal attributions, and generalizability of results.

Validity in Evaluation

In this section the validity types are discussed in greater detail and their implications for quantitative public health research practice are considered. For each validity issue, Cook and Campbell identify "threats" to validity, alternative explanations for the assertion that a particular study or finding is actually representative of the true condition.

Statistical Conclusion Validity

This discussion should be framed within the logic of type 1 and type 2 errors and examined in the context of a practical and realistic example, such as educational programs to prevent HIV infection among adolescents (Kirby et al., 1994). (The evaluation problem of this example is modeled after a recently published report by O'Hara et al., 1996.) Suppose that baseline (e.g., pretest) data concerning a set of relevant outcome indicators (e.g., HIV knowledge, skills to identify and deflect or avoid unwanted sexual situations, and intentions to use condoms) are collected from high school students. A multicomponent educational intervention is then presented to the students, and measurements of exposure (e.g., in hours of classroom time) are made. One school year later, a follow-up (e.g., posttest) survey on the identical outcomes is administered.

The question posed by statistical conclusion validity for this example is: "Does the sample show a relationship between exposure to the educational intervention and changes in the outcomes as measured by scores on a battery of items measuring HIV knowledge, skills in identification of 'risky' social situations, and condom use intentions?" Suppose a relationship between exposure and positive changes in knowledge, skills, and intentions was found. What kinds of errors could be made in inferring that such a positive relationship exists between the HIV education intervention and the outcomes? The possibilities should be considered assuming that the actual efficacy of the intervention in increasing preventive behaviors related to HIV infection is known, as shown in Table 9.1 (Wonnacott and Wonnacott, 1987; Gonick and Smith, 1993).

Note that the data on the relationship between exposure and outcome (represented by the "Yes" row of Table 9.1) alone are not totally persuasive. The intervention may have been unrelated to change in knowledge or intentions. This situation is reflected by the Yes/No cell in the top row, a type 1 error, or a false-positive when the "truth" is compared with the sample result; statisticians would call this an "alpha" error represented by α (see Chapter 2). Usually the probability for a false-positive is set at 1 chance in 20 (0.05) for reasons that are both historical and statistical (Cowles and Davis, 1982).

Of course, the opposite logical mistake also could be made. Suppose that in the sample no relationship is found between exposure and preventive skill acquisition, although in actuality, HIV prevention education has a positive influence on such skills. This mistake is the reverse of the previous one: it is a type 2 error, or a false-negative, when the "truth" is compared with the sample result. This error is labeled a "beta" error represented by β. In summary, the essence of assessing statistical conclusion validity is increased by minimizing risk of type 1 and type 2 errors.

Threats to Statistical Conclusion Validity

In the case of statistical conclusion validity, threats to validity are causes of making type 1 and type 2 errors. Two major errors are relevant here. The first is *low statistical power,* the ability of the study to detect real differences in samples of observations. When the goal of evaluations is to detect minimal differences or as-

Table 9.1 Truth: Exposure to Intervention Is Associated with Positive Preventive Outcomes

		Yes	*No*
Do we find such a relationship in the sample?	Yes	Accurate Inference	Type 1 error, or a false-positive
	No	Type 2 error, or a false-negative	Accurate Inference

sociations, determining the statistical power of a study during the design phase is important.

Continuing with the example of making type 1 or type 2 errors in assessing the relationship between program exposure and preventive skill acquisiton, the assertion that exposure to HIV education and the relevant outcomes are related should not be rejected merely because the research plan is successful in identifying only substantial, but not subtle, associations. Suppose that the intervention had a minimal effect on knowledge, skills, and intentions, representing only a 2% increase in skill as classroom hours of exposure increased. If an evaluation design were used that could reliably detect increases of only 20% in skills, we would make the erroneous assertion that HIV education and exposure were unrelated (a type 2 error). An association between HIV education and cognitive or behavioral outcomes is important—even if it is as subtle as implied in this example.

The second important threat to validity is *measurement error.* Measures with high proportions of random error also can provide very poor estimates of associations, leading to findings of no relationship when a relationship would have been uncovered if the measures were less error prone. Statistical approaches can be used to minimize measurement error. For example, unstandardized regression coefficients are less sensitive to measurement error in the dependent variable than correlations or standardized regression coefficients (Greenland et al., 1986; Wonnacott and Wonnacott, 1987). In summary, measures composed of a high proportion of random error tend to produce type 2 errors leading to the false conclusion that the variables of interest are not assǫciated when the truth is otherwise.

Type 2 errors are common in standard evaluation designs. For example, Rossi (1990), Lipsey (1990), and Grimes and Schulz (1996) conclude that most empirical studies in educational, public health, and clinical research were insensitive to minimal associations. In an evaluation context, this means that some evaluation studies report "no difference" or "no effect" of the treatments because of low statistical power independent of the actual efficacy of the interventions under scrutiny. These false-negative results reflect the influence of type 2 errors.

Reducing Threats to Statistical Conclusion Validity

Both of these threats to validity have solutions. Often, low statistical power is inappropriately "designed into" the evaluation study through oversight. However, simple personal computer programs can estimate power given different assumptions concerning the sample size, variability in the outcome variable, and the size of the effect to be detected (e.g., POWER and EPI-INFO). In addition, many statistical texts have extensive user friendly discussions of statistical power that include the formulas to compute power and sample size for a comprehensive range of potential evaluation designs that may include cluster sampling and repeated measurements (e.g., Motulsky, 1995; Murray and Hannan, 1990). Thus, only a basic understanding of the principles involved is necessary to estimate these important parameters of the proposed research.

Construct Validity

Construct validity is concerned with the meanings or labels researchers attach to the empirical measures they use and addresses whether the evaluation design allows for meaningful measures and scales. The basic tool for the quantitative determination of construct validity is the measurement model, one component of a broad class of statistical analysis known as *structural equation modeling* (Hoyle and Smith, 1994) (Fig. 9.1). In such analyses, unobserved constructs are shown in circles and observed measures ("indicators") are in rectangles (Hoyle and Panter, 1995). For example, in assessing the unobserved construct of self-efficacy toward a particular task (Bandura, 1992; Fishbein, 1997) such as consistent condom use to prevent HIV infection and other STDs (Lawrance et al., 1990; Wulfert and Wan, 1993) or the adoption of new personal health promotion activities (Grembowski et al., 1993), six observed variables might be the respondents' interval

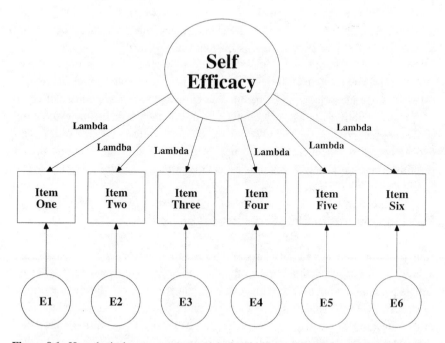

Figure 9.1. Hypothetical measurement model of self-efficacy. Measurement model types (1) Parallel—all lambdas equal, all error variances equal. (2) Tau-equivalent—different lambdas, all error variances equal. (3) Congeneric—different lambdas, different error variances.

rankings of their self-reported, self-efficacy toward condom use under many different social situations (e.g., when one of the partners is under the influence of alcohol) (Fig. 9.1). The small circles represent the unobserved measurement error terms of each of the observed variables. Finally, the single-headed arrows are the regression coefficients relating the observed variables and their unobserved causes.

Note that two sets of single-headed arrows are used—one set from the construct that reflects concept-caused variability of the observed data in rectangles and one set from the error terms of each of the indicators that reflect measurement error. Sometimes the arrows go from the indicators to the concepts, but these "causal indicator" models are different from the measurement model of Figure 9.1 (Cohen et al., 1990; MacCallum and Browne, 1993). Conceptually, this double pair of single-headed arrows implies that observed data items are a function of both concept-relevant and concept-irrelevant (e.g., measurement error) sources. This partitioning of an observed score into one component representing the construct and one reflecting error is the basic model for "true score" measurement theory (Traub, 1994). Ideally, the regression coefficients from the concepts to the indicators would be high and the coefficients from the measurement error terms would be minimal. The "reliability" of an individual measure is calculated as the ratio of variance from the construct divided by the total variance in the observed item (Streiner and Norman, 1995).

Reliability also can be defined for complete measurement models (e.g., Fig. 9.1). The specific formula, however, depends on the assumptions being made about both the concept-to-term regression coefficients linking the items to the construct and the measurement error variances of the items. Three patterns are commonly defined. *Parallel* measurement models assume that all construct-item coefficients are equal and that the item variance is also equal. *Tau-equivalent* measurement models assume equality of regression coefficients but not of error variances across the items. Finally, *congeneric* measurement models do not assume any necessary equality (Millsap and Everson, 1991). Of course, each measurement model is less restrictive than the one preceding it, and in each case, a formula exists for the reliability of the composite formed assuming one of the three types of measurement models (Reuterberg and Gustafsson, 1992).

Threats to Construct Validity

Measurement modeling can explicitly assess levels of random measurement error in both individual indicators and composite scales; proposed measures can then be refined to reduce measurement error. This refinement increases both statistical power (even holding constant sample size) and construct validity. Thus, measurement modeling reduces threats to two dimensions of validity simultaneously.

However, both question development and measurement modeling are technically complex, although Schuman and Presser (1996) provide an excellent introduction to the first task. Both tasks require small data sets to pretest and develop the initial measures before refinement. Thus in most cases, a superior approach is to use instruments that have been validated and well documented. Some collections of measures for public health researchers are now appearing (e.g., Card, 1993; Lorig et al., 1996). More of these collections should be compiled for a range of cognitive, behavioral, and clinical outcomes relevant to public health researchers.

Internal Validity

Internal validity is concerned with the assertion that the intervention actually caused the outcome, as opposed to some uncontrolled variable of the environment or characteristics of the respondents. Thus, internal validity is concerned with the important task of *assessing the plausibility* of causal claims. In the HIV-education example, a positive relationship between exposure and the outcome measures (in the absence of a type 1 error), usually leads to a causal claim that exposure to the intervention actually caused the increase.

As usual, threats to internal validity exist. Consider the research design as described:

Pretest	HIV education	Posttest
(Baseline)	(Intervention)	(Follow-up)

In this example, a positive relationship between exposure and outcome change was found in the sample of students who participated in the study, using a *t*-test of the difference between pretest and posttest means or a regression analysis with hours of classroom exposure as the independent variable. Both analyses were corrected for the repeated measure design (i.e., the same respondents are surveyed at two time points, and thus the observations are not independent). However, evaluators typically want more than just confidence in their statistical conclusions; they want to be able to say that the HIV education intervention *caused* the observed relationship between exposure and the increase in knowledge, skills, and intention.

What are some alternatives to this causal assertion (i.e., what are the threats to internal validity in this example?) One likely alternative might be *maturation* (i.e., students may acquire skills or knowledge from the process of growing up and encountering different social situations). Thus, the true explanation for the apparent efficacy of the intervention is that students "naturally" become more self-assured and socially proficient with age, regardless of the intervention program itself.

Another common threat in this context is *testing:* improvement on the posttest because of taking the pretest. To eliminate the alternative explanation of practice effects, the administrators might switch the test forms at the posttest, exactly in anticipation of the testing effect discussed above. But suppose the posttest was now easier than the previous one, so again it appears that the students improve over time (this is the threat of *instrumentation* where changes in survey items are misinterpreted for the effect of the intervention). A solution to both of these problems is the development of "parallel forms" of tests (i.e., sets of items that are equivalently difficult but also meaningfully different). Suppose that the posttest has different items but is equally difficult (i.e., both testing and instrumentation are eliminated as a threat to internal validity). Again, however, there might be a problem. In this case, students who liked the program may have attended all the sessions, and students who did not like it may have been erratic in attendance. This threat to validity would be *selection* resulting from attrition.

All these scenarios make a general point. These potential threats to internal validity (and other threats that were not mentioned) are alternative explanations for the assertion that exposure to the HIV-education intervention caused the positive performances on the outcomes. In all cases, the intervention is legitimately associated with skills—the results are high in terms of statistical conclusion validity. The HIV-education program, however, is not the cause of this association. In the case of maturation, for example, the observed association is due to the natural improvement in social skills (including avoiding sexually risky situations) associated with age, which creates an appearance that the intervention program caused the increased performance on the posttest.

Threats to Internal Validity

The classical solution to most of the threats to internal validity is the *randomized clinical trial* (RCT). (RCTs are usually called "randomized experiments" in evaluation studies). The advantage of the RCT lies in the constitution of the groups to be exposed to the intervention or experimental treatment on the basis of chance or *randomization.* Thus, by using a rule for allocation that is unpredictable, groups usually are equivalent or comparable before they are exposed to the intervention. Because of this initial equivalence, if outcome differences (i.e., treatment effects) are statistically detected (i.e., high statistical conclusion validity), they must be caused by the operation or processes of the intervention, because differential treatment exposure is the only way in which the groups were different at the outset.

However, RCTs do not eliminate all threats to internal validity (Cook and Campbell, 1979). For example, differential subject attrition over time may systematically undermine the initial equivalency of the treatment and control groups. However, statistical tests are useful in identifying such attrition and *selection bias modeling* can be used to adjust for these breakdowns of the randomization process (Foster and Bickman, 1996; Berk et al., 1988).

In addition, the implementation of RCTs often is not feasible in public health. For example, a randomized clinical trial to assess the impacts of changes in nursing-home restraint practices described previously could not be conducted because all nursing homes are affected by the new statutes; implementing the new regulations in some nursing homes and maintaining the original regulations in others cannot be done on a random basis. Thus, *quasi-experimental designs* (research designs that do not utilize random assignment to deliberately construct an initial equivalence between groups) often are used.

Some types of quasi-experiments are higher in internal validity than others. For example, in the *regression discontinuity design* (Trochim, 1989), the assignment to treatment and control status is not made on the basis of randomization (as for the RCT) but on the basis of a known, quantitative rule. Of course, if the assignment rule effectively differentiates between the units assigned, the experimental groups are constituted differently before exposure to the treatment interventions. But as long as the assignment rule was the only basis on which the units were differentially assigned to treatment/control status, statistical adjustments can be made during the analysis of the data to estimate unbiased treatment effects. This design has been used in educational interventions where ethical justifications prevail for assigning students who "need the intervention" to experimental programs and students who "don't need the intervention" to status quo teaching methods.

While the regression discontinuity design seems "fairer" than RCTs in many research contexts, implementation is complicated by the difficulty of the construction of an appropriate assignment rule acceptable to all parties and universally applied to all cases. Note also that as in any controlled trial, "cheating" on the assignment destroys the ability to remove statistically the initial nonequivalency of the two groups and thus leads to biased treatment effects.

In addition, regression discontinuity designs are often impossible or unrealistic for some evaluation problems. For policy experiments, other types of quasi-experiments [e.g., series *interrupted time series* (Horn and Heerboth, 1982)] that compare outcomes before and after the policy change (e.g., Rock, 1992) can also be persuasive, especially if outcomes are combined with data from other units where the policy change has not taken place. For example, states' policies toward drinking and driving may vary. A policy change lowering the blood alcohol level defining intoxication may be evaluated using data collected before and after the law change in one state combined with data from other states where the intoxication level did not change. If the "treatment" state shows reductions in alcohol-related crash mortality, the alternative hypothesis of maturation (or "secular trend") is eliminated if the comparison states showed no decline over the same time period.

The change in the approach to the interpretation when RCTs are not possible and quasi-experiments are substituted in their place should be noted. Usually, specific design features must be instituted to eliminate each alternative explanation separately when quasi-experiments are used. Interpretation of quasi-experimental results is problematic, because some threats to internal validity often are impossible to completely "design away." The evaluator's role in this case is to anticipate and compensate for likely threats to internal validity in the proposed research design while discounting other threats through logical argument rather than design features (Cordray, 1986). This task is obviously more difficult than relying on the power of randomization to produce high levels of internal validity, because the clever critic always can propose an alternative explanation to explain the results of quasi-experiments that were not considered by the original researchers. Thus, quasi-experiments usually have lower internal validity than RCTs.

External Validity

External validity defines the researcher's ability to generalize to other persons, places, and times. Often, the concern in relation to a particular study is the "representativeness" of the persons, subjects, or times sampled or reported. Evaluations also use other sampling strategies. First, results should be generalizable to specific target populations of policy interest and not necessarily the general population (e.g., the working poor, released prisoners with no history of mental instability or drug abuse, children from educationally disadvantaged environments, the homeless, or adolescents at risk for STD infection). Even before the study takes places, the researcher should have some idea of the populations of interest.

Other aspects of "generalizability" relevant for narrowly defined groups are important. For example, generalizing across populations might be a concern of a health educator who wishes to design an intervention program. Data may suggest that a particular health promotion intervention works for economically disadvantaged rural residents in North Carolina; but will this intervention work for similar populations on Indian reservations or for Hispanic adolescents in New Mexico?

External validity can be improved by using appropriate sampling approaches (Cook and Campbell, 1979). First, *sampling for representativeness* best reflects the conventional wisdom found in standard survey research texts. When the researcher defines the relevant population, takes simple random samples, and tries to ensure high response rates, generalizations to the larger population can be made (see Chapter 2).

Alternatives to sampling for representativeness are often used in evaluation studies that are attractive when numerically small populations of high epidemiological or public health importance are of particular interest. For example, to select large numbers of persons at risk for HIV infection from injecting drug use (Anderson et al., 1996) or to locate African Americans at risk for heart disease

(Bertram, 1994), simple random sampling would be logistically complicated, extremely expensive, and wasteful of all the observations that were not ultimately utilized.

In such cases, *sampling for modal instances,* similar to quota sampling, might be more appropriate. For example, school systems have limited resources and many are able to implement an experimental program for HIV prevention in only a few schools. Which schools should they choose? A random sample of schools tends to result in types of schools that are most common in the district. An alternative is to select one unit from each of some typology of school types (e.g., mostly minority, mixed student composition, and mostly majority). The task is to find a single school that represents the "average" school in each school type, a problem that random sampling of schools would certainly not solve. The HIV-education program would be implemented in each of the three "average" schools of each type.

Another appropriate alternative to the classical sampling for representativeness model is *sampling for heterogeneity.* For assessment of programs, this type of sampling is often beneficial because it is rare to repeat studies more than once. Thus, to assess the effects of programs across contexts and target populations, it may make sense to purposively sample a range of settings and target groups, even if they represent demographically unrepresentative groups and statistically unlikely (albeit policy-relevant) social contexts. To the statistician, the identification of populations that are maximally similar within grouping and maximally dissimilar between grouping is remarkably like the functions of cluster analysis, a method for quantitatively arriving at heterogenous but meaningful groupings of sample units (Van Ryzin, 1995).

Threats to External Validity

Assessing external validity depends more on the ultimate purpose of the evaluation than any of the three other threats. "Policy-relevant representativeness" may demand the selection of units for observations that would be considered quite unrepresentative using the logic of textbook sampling approaches. In evaluation contexts, producing widely generalizable estimates of program effects is of limited interest, largely because the need to generalize the effective programs often is minimal. This issue raises the topic of the interrelationships between the validity types and their priorities within a scientific hierarchy of values, a topic discussed in the case study example and revisited briefly in the conclusion.

Application of the Validity Assessment: Project RESPECT

Although validity type assessments normally are used as diagnostic instruments for comparing competing evaluation research plans, they can also be used retrospectively to examine particular evaluation projects. A recently completed multi-site randomized trial of three different modalities of counseling and testing for HIV and other STD infection (Project RESPECT) illustrates the four validity types.

Description of Interventions

In Project RESPECT investigators compared three separate HIV/STD prevention interventions as part of a randomized controlled trial of HIV-negative persons. These interventions were an informational intervention, *HIV education,* and two other different counseling interventions—-*HIV prevention counseling,* and *enhanced HIV prevention counseling.* Each of the three interventions focused on achieving a single behavior—consistent condom use during sexual intercourse with primary and/or other sex partners. For all three interventions in an STD clinic, each succeeding counseling session built on the previous sessions and used an HIV pretest and posttest protocol. Session 1 always included a discussion of the test. Test results were given from 7 to 10 days later (during session 2 for HIV education and HIV prevention counseling), or in session 3 for enhanced HIV prevention counseling. A brief description of each type of counseling follows.

The *HIV education* intervention consisted of two 5 minute informational sessions about preventing STDs and HIV. The pretest message was given by the clinician (medical practitioner), who examined and treated the study participant for STDs during the initial clinic visit. The message included information about the HIV test and prevention information relevant to the participant's reported risk behaviors. The posttest session took place 7 to 10 days later when the participant returned for the HIV test results. During the posttest session, the clinician or counselor informed the participant about the test results and the limitations of the test, again using a didactic approach and not engaging the participant in an interactive counseling process. HIV transmission risks were reiterated, and specific behaviors or circumstances that placed the participant at risk for acquiring HIV or other STDs were identified again.

In response to concern that true *HIV prevention counseling* was not occurring in STD clinics and with advice from experts on counseling theory and practice, in 1993 the Centers for Disease Control and Prevention (CDC) recommended a client-centered HIV-prevention counseling model for use in all U.S. STD clinics (CDC, 1993, 1994). Project RESPECT's HIV prevention counseling intervention differed from CDC's model only in its focus on condom use rather than on a wider variety of HIV/STD risk behaviors. The intervention consisted of two 20 minute, client-focused, interactive counseling sessions with an HIV counselor. The first (i.e., pretest) session took place at the initial clinic visit before the STD examination, and the second (posttest) session occurred 7 to10 days later, when the HIV test results returned. The counseling sessions focused on each participant's highest

HIV/STD risk or greatest concern. The pretest session concluded with a behavioral goal-setting exercise in which the participant arrived at a small behavioral risk-reduction step that he or she could make before the final posttest session.

The multisession *enhanced HIV prevention counseling* intervention was based on the theory of reasoned action (Fishbein et al., 1991), other psychosocial concepts, and the health-belief model. This intervention consisted of four interactive counseling sessions with an HIV counselor. The first session took place during the initial clinic visit before the clinical examination and lasted 20 minutes (this session was identical to the first HIV counseling session described previously). The remaining sessions took place over the following 3 weeks, each session lasting 60 minutes. The sessions in this intervention attempted to change key theoretical variables underlying the decision to use (or not to use) condoms. In the first session of enhanced HIV prevention counseling (which was identical to the first session of HIV prevention counseling) the HIV counselor helped participants assess their own risks for HIV and STDs, identified barriers to reducing risks, and arrived at an achievable first step toward changing risk through the use of condoms. During session 2, the focus was on changing attitudes toward condom use. During session 3, the focus was on changing self-efficacy for using condoms. The main focus of the session was directed at increasing self-efficacy; that is, one's belief that one can consistently use (or get one's partner to use) a condom. The focus of session 4 was exploring community norms and social support for consistent condom use. The session ended with the participant arriving at a long-term strategy for behavior change toward the goal of consistent condom use.

Respondents and Variables

Project RESPECT enrolled persons (2440 men and 1860 women) into one of the three intervention groups. All enrolled persons self-identified as heterosexual completed baseline interviews; postintervention data were obtained through interviews conducted immediately following the final intervention session (the "immediate follow-up") and through interviews conducted at four scheduled visits (at 3, 6, 9, and 12 months after enrollment). Project RESPECT's intervention completion rates were high. Overall, 82% of participants completed all of their assigned intervention sessions; 72% completed all four sessions of the *enhanced HIV prevention counseling* intervention (most of the attrition came after the first session), 86% completed both sessions of the *HIV prevention counseling* intervention, and 85% completed both sessions of the *HIV education* intervention. Intervention completion overall varied slightly among men (80%) and women (83%); the higher completion rate among women occurred regardless of intervention type.

Data were collected on outcome (HIV and STD risk behaviors), determinants as a means of increasing the employee's commitment to goals or as a means of increasing acceptance for new job procedures, the employee becomes more interested in information about how he is doing. As a result, feedback on job performance becomes an extremely important part of motivation.

Knowledge of Results

As was pointed out in Chapter XII, it is essential to provide knowledge of performance results in a regular and timely manner in order to increase and sustain high levels of motivation. Regular knowledge of results has proven to be of value from both informational and motivational points of

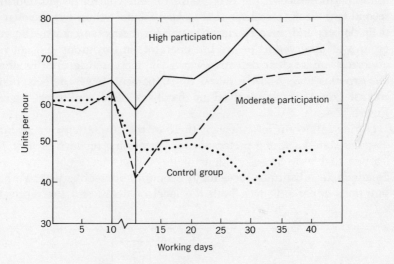

Figure 13.3   Relationship between participation and performance, adapted from (A. Marrow, *Industrial Psychology Pays in This Plan, loc. cit.*).

view. Before any improvement in performance can be expected, an employee must be informed of his past performance and be given specific suggestions for the kinds of improvements that are expected. In addition, feedback which indicates an individual is performing up to expectations, or is improving, can be an excellent means of sustaining motivation. Even when feedback indicates that performance is not up to expectations, it can provide an opportunity for employee motivation if the supervisor approaches the situation with a positive attitude. One means of accomplishing this is to indicate confidence in the employee's ability to achieve the desired goal and to concentrate on determining what type of assistance the employee needs to raise his performance to the desired level.

Although the value of feedback has been demonstrated in a number of laboratory and educational settings, only a limited number of studies has investigated the impact of knowledge of results in an industrial setting. Several recent studies at Autonetics, however, have confirmed the value of feeding back performance data to assembly personnel. One study investigated the extent to which feedback of defect information would improve performance of electronic assemblers [12]. A control group of seven operators and an experimental group of 13 operators were matched in terms of previous experience and prior performance level. Both groups were observed for a two-week period during which neither group was provided with a significant amount of feedback. There was no difference in the performance of the two groups for this control period. During the second two weeks members of the experimental group were shown all of their defects and were required to correct their own errors. The control group was observed as before but operators in this group did not review or correct any of their defective work. The increased level of feedback in the experimental group resulted in 70 percent fewer defects than the control group which received no feedback. The results are shown in Figure 13.4.

During follow-up interviews with 15 of the 20 participants all but one operator stated a strong preference for performing his own rework. It was learned that written descriptions of the defects were not considered to be adequate substitutes for actually seeing the defective part. Verbal descriptions apparently lack both the level of detail and the motivational

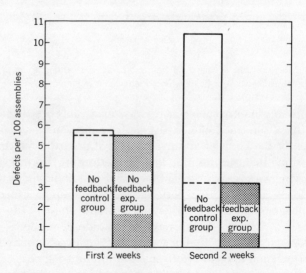

Figure 13.4   The effect of knowledge-of-results on electronic assembly performance.

value that is obtained from seeing and reworking the actual hardware defect. As a result of these findings and experience gained from conducting similar studies, the following recommendations were provided for effective feedback systems: (a) when a defective part is identified, it should be returned as soon as possible to the responsible manufacturing supervisor or leadman, (b) the supervisor should discuss each defect with the operator who produced it and make a specific recommendation for avoiding such errors in the future, (c) each operator should be allowed to perform his own rework, and (d) to provide a means of controlling feedback, random samples of rework items should be examined each week to determine what percentage is *actually* being returned to the original operator for rework.

In addition to rapid feedback of information on performance, some form of recognition for achievement is required to sustain high levels of motivation.

Recognition for Achievement

Perhaps one of the easiest but most neglected means of sustaining motivation is to provide recognition for achievement. Unfortunately many supervisors are so busy that their only contact with employees usually involves areas where improvement is required. Even when constructive criticism is provided, a continual pattern of critical comments rather than recognition for accomplishment will lead to decreased motivation. Recognition is a powerful form of motivation because it provides tangible evidence that extra effort is really worthwhile. Recognition is particularly effective when it is provided in a form of more interesting assignments, increased responsibility, deserved promotions, and merited pay increases.

One of the most essential steps in assuring effective recognition or reward practices is for the company to make sure that the rewards provided are really the ones that are most generally desired by employees [13]. Although this seems like an obvious and simple step, few companies have used techniques such as modern attitude measurement to improve the effectiveness of their reward practices. As a result many of our recognition practices may seem to be highly valued by management but have little if any effect on the average worker. The systematic determination of optimum reward practices is especially important in developing and administering employee pay practices.

Economic Incentives

The importance of money as a source of motivation depends largely on what the money represents to a person; money should not be regarded as a universal motivator. One of the primary problems in understanding the

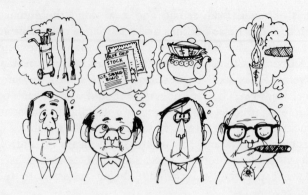

value of money is that it is a symbol that represents different things to different people. It can serve to satisfy needs such as achievement, prestige, or security because it can be a measure of success, status, or protection. However, employees often leave higher paying jobs for others that are more interesting and provide a greater challenge. Other individuals may choose to remain in a secure low-paying job rather than risk an increase in pay with more responsibility and more chance of failure. As a result, we must conclude that the effect of money is highly dependent on what it represents to each individual.

In general, salary increases which are based on merit and other forms of pay which symbolize achievement have a high degree of motivational value. However, general pay increases, group insurance plans, and many other types of standard economic benefits which apply equally to all individuals in a company have little, if any, long-term motivational value. In fact, any type of economic benefit that becomes automatic or tends to increase at regular intervals is of little motivational value and may easily become a source of dissatisfaction if employee expectations are not met.

An effective technique for using money as a motivator is to tie salary increases to the accomplishment of some specific objectives. In this system the supervisor and the employee jointly develop the subordinate's objectives for the next six months or year. It is extremely important to both parties to agree on exactly how progress toward these goals is to be measured and what types or amounts of reward are to be given for various levels of achievement. At the end of the agreed-on period both men should jointly participate in determining the progress and establishing new goals for the next period. Unfortunately, this type of practice is generally limited to management and sales positions. Most first line supervisors are severely restricted in terms of the freedom that they have to determine type and amount of rewards that their employees will receive.

Because of the factors outlined, we should not rely on financial rewards as a primary means of motivating employees. Effective pay practices,

Suggested Readings

Program Evaluation

Campbell, D. T. Methods for the experimenting society. *Eval. Pract.* 12 :223–260, 1991.

This is an expanded version of the article originally published in 1969. It is arguably the most influential work to affect quantitative evaluation procedures. It also has an extensive and thoughtful discussion of analyzing the threats to validity, which are discussed only briefly above.

Pirie, P., E. Stone, A. Assaf, J. Flora, and U. Maschewsky-Schneider. Program evaluation strategies for community-based health promotion programs: perspectives from the cardiovascular disease community research and demonstration studies. *Health Educ. Res.* 9:23–36, 1994.

Cook and Campbell's validity types are not the only criteria for retrospectively assessing evaluation studies. This article compares four large community interventions on the basis of eight dimensions: formative research, quality assurance, delivered dose of intervention, received dose of intervention, intervention component impact, intermediate impact, community impact, and cost analysis.

Shadish, W. R., T. D. Cook, and L. C. Leviton. *Foundations of Program Evaluation.* Newbury Park, CA: Sage Publications.

This is an intellectual and historical review of the founders of evaluation: Scriven, Campbell, Weiss, Wholey, Stake, Cronbach, and Rossi. It is indispensable.

Wholey, J. S., H. P. Hatry, and K. E. Newcomer. *Handbook of Practical Program Evaluation.* San Francisco, CA: Jossey-Bass, 1994.

An up-to-date selection of different chapters devoted to problem solving in evaluation.

Randomized Clinical Trials

Friedman, L. M., C. D. Furberg, and D. L. DeMets. *Fundamentals of Clinical Trials.* Littleton, MA: PSG Publishing Company, 1985.

Selection Bias Modeling

Dubin, J. A., and D. Rivers. Selection bias in linear regression, logit, and probit models. *Sociol. Meth. Res.* 18:360–390, 1989.

Haveman, R. H. Methods for correcting selectivity bias: a legacy of war on poverty research. *Sociol. Soc. Res.* 71:4–10, 1986.

Reynolds, A. J., and J. A. Temple. Quasi-experimental estimates of the effects of a preschool intervention: psychometric and econometric comparisons. *Eval. Rev.* 19: 347–373, 1995.

Rindskopf, D. New developments in selection modeling for quasi-experimentation. In *Advances in Quasi-experimental Design and Analysis. New Directions in Program Evaluation #31,* edited by W. M. Trochim. San Francisco, CA: Jossey-Bass, 1986, pp. 79–89.

Winship, C., and R. D. Mare. Models for sample selection bias. *Annu. Rev. Sociol.* 18: 327–350, 1992.

Quasi-Experiments

Cappelleri, J. C., W. M. Trochim, T. D. Stanley, and C. S. Reichardt. Random measurement error does not bias the treatment effect estimates in the regression-discontinuity design: the case of no interaction. *Eval. Rev.* 154:395–419, 1991.

Grossman, J., and J. P. Tierney. The fallibility of comparison groups. *Eval. Rev.* 175: 556–571, 1993.

Mohr, L. B. *Impact Analysis for Program Evaluation.* Thousand Oaks, CA: Sage Publications, 1995.

Trochim, W. M., J. C. Cappelleri, and C. S. Reichardt. Random measurement error does not bias the treatment effect estimates in the regression-discontinuity design: when an interaction effect is present. *Eval. Rev.* 155:571–604, 1991.

Structural Equation Modeling

Bentler, P. M., and J. A. Stein. Structural equation models in medical research. *Stat. Meth. Med. Res.* 1:159–181, 1992. *An overview of how SEM can be applied to common research problems in medical and public health research.*

Bollen, K., and R. Lennox. Conventional wisdom on measurement: a structural equation perspective. *Psychol. Bull.* 1102:305–314, 1991. *A discussion of how standard measurement theory can be subsumed under the general SEM approach.*

Schumacker, R. E., and R. G. Lomax. *A Beginner's Guide to Structural Equation Modeling.* Mahwah, NJ: Lawrence Erlbaum, 1996. *An excellent introduction to the elements of structural equation modeling (e.g., path analysis, measurement models, determining goodness-of fit, comparing models across respondent groups)].*

References

Anderson, J. C., and D. W. Gerbing. Structural equation modeling in practice: a review and recommended two-step approach. *Psychol. Bull.* 103:411–423, 1988.

Anderson, J. E., R. Cheney, M. Clatts, et al. HIV risk behavior, street outreach, and condom use in eight high-risk populations. *AIDS Educ. Prev.* 8:191–204, 1996.

Aral, S.O., and T. A. Peterman. Measuring outcomes of behavioral interventions for STD/HIV prevention. *Int. J. STD AIDS* 7(Suppl.):30–38, 1996.

Bandura, A. A social cognitive approach to the exercise of control over AIDS infection. In: *Adolescents and AIDS,* edited by R. J. DiClemente. Newbury Park, CA: Sage Publications, 1992.

Berk, R. A., and P. H. Rossi. *Thinking about Program Evaluation.* Newbury Park, CA: Sage Publications, 1990.

Berk, R. A., G. K. Smyth, and L. W. Sherman. When random assignment fails: some lessons from the Minneapolis spouse abuse experiment. *J. Quant. Criminol.* 4: 209–223, 1988.

Bertram, D. A pilot study to estimate the cost of a telephone survey of rare populations: African Americans and persons with angina. *Eval. Rev.* 186:718–729, 1994.

Bollen, K., and R. Lennox. Conventional wisdom on measurement: a structural equation perspective. *Psychol. Bull.* 1102:305–314, 1991.

Brown, R. L., and B. L. Carlson. Early diagnosis of substance abuse: evaluation of a course of computer-assisted instruction. *Med. Educ.* 245:438–446, 1990.

Campbell, D. T. Relabeling internal and external validity for applied social scientists. In: *Advances in Quasi-experimental Design and Analysis. New Directions in Program Evaluation #31,* edited by W. M. Trochin. San Francisco, CA: Jossey-Bass, 1986, pp. 31:67–77.

Campbell, D. T., and J. C. Stanley. *Experimental and Quasi-experimental Designs for Research.* Chicago, IL: Rand McNally, 1966.

Card, J. J. *Handbook of Adolescent Sexuality and Pregnancy: Research and Evaluation Instruments.* Newbury Park, CA: Sage Publications, 1993.

Casswell, S., L. Stewart, and P. Duignan. The struggle against the broadcast of anti-health messages: regulation of alcohol advertising in New Zealand 1980–1987. *Health Promot.* 4:287–296, 1989.

Centers for Disease Control and Prevention. Technical guidance on HIV counseling. *MMWR Morb. Mortal. Wkly. Rep.* 42:11–17, 1993.

Centers for Disease Control and Prevention. *HIV Counseling, Testing, and Referral Standards and Guidelines.* Atlanta, GA: U.S. Department of Health and Human Services, 1994.

Chen, H.-T. *Theory Driven Evaluations.* Newbury Park, CA: Sage Publications, 1990.

Cohen, P., J. Cohen, J. Teresi, M. Marchi, and C. N. Velez. Problems in the measurement of latent variables in structural equation causal models. *Appl. Psychol. Measurement* 14:183–196, 1990.

Cook, T. D., and D. T. Campbell. *Quasi-experimentation: Design and Analysis Issues for Field Settings.* Chicago, IL: Rand McNally, 1979.

Cordray, D. S. Quasi-experimental analysis: a mixture of methods and judgment. *Advances in Quasi-experimental Design and Analysis. New Directions for Program Evaluation, #31,* edited by W. M. Trochim. San Francisco, CA: Jossey-Bass, 1986.

Cowles, M., and C. Davis. On the origin of the .05 level of statistical significance. *Am. Psychol.* 37:553–558, 1982.

Cronbach, L. *Designing Evaluations of Educational and Social Programs.* San Francisco, CA: Jossey-Bass, 1982.

Dehar, M., S. Casswell, and P. Duignan. Formative and process evaluation of health promotion and disease prevention programs. *Eval. Rev.* 17:204–220, 1993.

Delewski, C., and R. F. Saltz. A community action approach to server intervention in two California counties. *Contemp. Drug Prob.* 345–368, 1990.

Demers, A., and L. Renaud. Formative evaluation of a nutritional marketing project in city-center restaurants. *Eval. Rev.* 16:634–649, 1992.

Dial, M. The misuse of evaluation in educational programs. In: *Preventing the Misuse of Evaluation. New Directions for Program Evaluation,* edited by C. J. Stevens, and M. Dial. San Francisco, CA: Jossey-Bass, 1994, pp. 61–67.

Diggle, P. J, K. Y. Liang, and S. L. Zeger. *Analysis of Longitudinal Data,* Oxford: Clarendon Press, 1995.

Dumka, L. E., M. W. Roosa, M. L. Michaels, and K .W. Suh. Using research and theory to develop prevention programs for high risk families. *Fam. Relations* 44:74–86, 1995.

Dunbar, J. M., R. R. Neufeld, H. C. White, and L. S. Libow. Retrain, don't restrain: the educational intervention of the national nursing home restraint removal project. *Gerontologist* 36: 539–542, 1996.

Fetterman, D. M. Empowerment evaluation. *Eval. Pract.* 15:1–15, 1994.

Finnegan, J., D. Murray, C. Kurth, and P. McCarthy. Measuring and tracking education program implementation: the Minnesota heart health program experience. *Health Educ. Q.* 16:77–90, 1989.

Fishbein, M., S. E. Middlestadt, and P. J. Hitchcock. Using information to change sexually transmitted disease-related behaviors: An analysis based on the theory of reasoned action. In: *Research Issues in Human Behavior and Sexually Transmitted Diseases in the AIDS Era,* edited by J. N. Wasserheit, et al. Washington, DC: American Society for Microbiology, 1991, pp. 243–257.

Fishbein, M. Predicting, understanding, and changing socially relevant behaviors: lessons learned. In: *The Message of Social Psychology,* edited by C. McGarty, and S. A. Haslam. Cambridge, MA: Blackwell, 1997, pp. 77–91.

Fitzpatrick, J. Roles of the evaluator in innovative programs. *Eval. Rev.* 12:449–461, 1988.

Fortmann, S. P., P. T. William, S. B. Hulley, N. Maccoby, and J. W. Farquhar. Does dietary health education reach only the privileged? *Circulation* 661:77–82, 1982.

Foster, E. M., and L. Bickman. An evaluator's guide to detecting attrition problems. *Eval. Rev.* 20:695–723, 1996.

Gonick, L., and W. Smith. *The Cartoon Guide to Statistics.* New York: Harper, 1993.

Graham, C. Exercise and aging: implications for persons with diabetes. *Diabetes Educ.* 17:189–195, 1991.

Green, L., and F. Lewis. *Measurement and Evaluation in Health Education and Health Promotion.* Palo Alto, CA: Mayfield Publishing, 1986.

Greenland, S., J. J. Schlesselman, and M. H. Criqui. The fallacy of employing standardized regression coefficients and correlations as measures of effect. *Am. J. Epidemiol.* 23:203–208,1986.

Grembowski, D., D. Patrick, P. Diehr, M. Durham, S. Beresford, E. Kay, and J. Hecht. Self-efficacy and health behavior among older adults. *J. Health Soc. Behav.* 34: 89–104, 1993.

Grimes, D. A., and K. F. Schulz. Determining sample size and power in clinical trials: the forgotten essential. *Semin. Reprod. Endocrinol.* 14:125–131, 1996.

Guba, E., and Y. Lincoln. *Fourth Generation Evaluation.* Newbury Park, CA: Sage Publications, 1989.

Hampson, S. E., R. E. Glasgow, and L. S. Foster. Personal models of diabetes among older adults: relationship of self-management and other variables. *Diabetes Educ.* 21: 300–307, 1995.

Hansen, W. B. School-based substance abuse prevention: a review of the state of the art in curriculum, 1980–1990. *Health Educ. Res.* 7:403–430, 1992.

Hausman, A., H. Spivak, D. Prothrow-Smith, and J. Roeber. Patterns of teen exposure to a community-based violence prevention project. *Adolesc. Health* 13:668–675, 1992.

Hennessy, C. H., and M. Hennessy. Community-based long term care for the elderly: evaluation practice reconsidered. *Med. Care Rev.* 47:221–259, 1990.

Hennessy, M., and M. Sullivan. Good organizational reasons for bad evaluation research. *Eval. Pract.* 10:41–50, 1989.

Hennessy, M. What works in program evaluation. *Eval. Pract.* 16:275–278, 1995.

Hennessy, M., and C. Grella. Evaluating innovative programs for homeless persons: case study of an unsuccessful proposal. *Eval. Pract.* 13:15–25, 1992.

Holder, H. D., R. F. Saltz, A. J. Treno, J. W. Grube, and R. B. Voas. Evaluation design for a community prevention trial. *Eval. Rev.* 21:140–165, 1997.

Horn, W., and J. Heerboth. Single case experimental designs and program evaluation. *Eval. Rev.* 6:403–442, 1982.

Hoyle, R. H., and G. T. Smith. Formulating clinical research hypotheses as structural equation models: a conceptual overview. *J. Consult. Clin. Psych.* 62:429–440, 1994.

Hoyle, R. H., and A. T. Panter. Writing about structural equation models. In: *Structural Equation Modeling: Concepts, Issues, and Applications,* edited by R. H. Hoyle. Thousand Oaks, CA.: Sage Publications, 1995.

Kamb, M. L., B. A. Dillon, M. Fishbein, and K. L. Willis. Quality assurance of HIV prevention counseling in a multi-center randomized controlled trial. *Public Health Rep.* 111(Suppl.):S99–S107, 1996.

Kaskutas, L., P. Morgan, and P. Vaeth. Structural impediments in the development of a community-based drug prevention program for youth. *Int. Q. Commun. Health Educ.* 12:169–182, 1991–92.

Kennedy, M. The role of the in-house evaluator. *Eval. Rev.* 7:519–541, 1983.

Kirby, D., L. Short, J. Collins, et al. School-based programs to reduce sexual risk behaviors: a review of effectiveness. *Public Health Rep.* 109:339–360, 1994.

Lawrance, L., S. R. Levy, and L. Rubinson. Self-efficacy and AIDS prevention for pregnant teens. *J. School Health* 60:19–24, 1990.

Leviton, L. C., and R. O. Valdiserri. Evaluating AIDS prevention: outcome, implementation, and mediating variables. *Eval. Prog. Plan.* 13:55–66,1990.

Lipsey, M. Theory as method: small theories of treatments. In:*New Directions in Program Evaluation #57,* edited by L. Sechrest, and A. Scott. San Francisco, CA: Jossey-Bass, 1993, pp. 5–38.

Lipsey, M. *Design Sensitivity.* Newbury Park, CA: Sage Publications, 1990.

Lorig, K., A. Stewart, P. Ritter, V. Gonzalez, D. Laurent, and J. Lynch. *Outcome Measures for Health Education and Other Health Care Interventions.* Newbury Park, CA: Sage Publications, 1996.

MacCallum, R. C., M. W. Browne. The use of causal indicators in covariance structure models: some practical issues. *Psychol. Bull.* 114:533–541, 1993.

McClintock, C. Evaluators as applied theorists. *Eval. Pract.* 11:1–12, 1990.

Middlestadt, S. E., K. Bhattacharyya, J. Rosenbaum, M. Fishbein, and M. Shepard. The use of theory based semistructured elicitation questionnaires: formative research for CDC's prevention marketing initiative. *Public Health Rep.* 111(Suppl.):S18–S27, 1996.

Millsap, R. E., and H. Everson. Confirmatory measurement model comparisons using latent means. *Multivariate Behav. Res.* 26:479–497, 1991.

Motulsky, H. *Intuitive Biostatistics.* New York: Oxford University Press, 1995.

Murray, D. M., and P. J. Hannan. Planning for the appropriate analysis in school-based drug-use prevention studies. *J. Consult. Clin. Psychol.* 58:458–468, 1990.

O'Hara, P., B. J. Messick, R. R. Fichtner, and D. Parris. A peer-led AIDS prevention program for students in an alternative school. *J. School Health* 66:176–182, 1996.

Pentz, M. A., C. Cormack, B. Flay, W. B. Hansen, and C. A. Johnson. Balancing program and research integrity in community drug abuse prevention: project STAR approach. *J. School Health.* 56:389–393, 1996.

Patton, M. Q. A world larger than formative or summative. *Eval. Pract.* 17:134–144, 1996.

Phillips, C. D., C. Hawes, and B. E. Fries. Reductions in the use of physical restraints in nursing homes: will it increase costs? *Am. J. Public Health* 83:342–348, 1993.

Reuterberg, S. E., and J. E. Gustafsson. Confirmatory factor analysis and reliability: testing measurement model assumptions. *Educ. Psychol. Measure.* 52:795–811, 1992.

Rock, S. M. Impact of the Illinois seat belt use law on accidents, deaths, and injuries. *Eval. Rev.* 16:491–507, 1992.

Ross, H. L. *Confronting drunk driving.* New Haven, CT: Yale University Press, 1992.

Rossi, J. S. Statistical power of psychological research: what have we gained in 20 years? *Consult. Clin. Psychol.* 58:646–656, 1990.

Rossi, P. H., and H. E. Freeman. *Evaluation: A Systematic Approach.* Thousand Oaks, CA: Sage Publications, 1993.

Saltz, R. F., P. J. Gruenewald, and M. Hennessy. Candidate alcohol problems and implications for measurement: general alcohol problems, outcome measures, instrumentation, and surrogates. In: *Community Prevention Trials for Alcohol Problems,* edited by H. D. Holder, and J. M. Howard, Westport, CT: Praeger Publishers, 1992.

Schuman, H., and S. Presser. *Questions and Answers in Attitude Surveys.* Thousand Oaks, CA: Sage Publications, 1996.

Scriven, M. Product evaluation: the state of the art. *Eval. Pract.* 15:45–62, 1994.

Short, L. M., and M. Hennessy. Using structural equations to estimate the effects of behavioral interventions. *Struct. Equat. Model.* 1:68–81, 1994.

Short, L. M., M. Hennessy, and J. Campbell. Tracking the work. In: *Family Violence: Building a Coordinated Community Response.* Chicago, IL: American Medical Association, 1996, pp. 59–72.

Smith, M. F. *Evaluability Assessment: A Practical Approach.* Boston: Kluwer Academic Publishers, 1989.

Steckler, A., R. M. Goodman, K. R. McLeroy, S. Davis, and G. Koch. Measuring the diffusion of innovative health promotion programs. *Am. J. Health Promot.* 6:214–224, 1992.

Streiner, D. L., and G. R. Norman. *Health Measurement Scales.* Oxford: Oxford University Press, 1995.

Traub, R. E. *Reliability for the Social Sciences.* Thousand Oaks, CA: Sage Publications, 1994.

Trochim, W. M. *Research Design for Program Evaluation: The Regression Discontinuity Approach.* Beverly Hills, CA: Sage Publications, 1989.

U.S. Preventive Services Task Force. Counseling to prevent HIV infection and other sexually transmitted diseases. In: *Guide to Clinical Preventive Services,* 2nd ed. Baltimore, MD: Williams & Wilkins, 1996, pp. 723–737.

Van Ryzin, G. G. Cluster analysis as a basis for purposive sampling of projects in case study evaluations. *Eval. Pract.* 16:109–119, 1995.

Wallack, L., and L. Dorfman. Media advocacy: a strategy for advancing policy and promoting health. *Health Educ. Q.* 23:293–317, 1996.

Wickizer, T. M., M. VonKorff, A. Cheadle, et al. Activating communities for health promotion: a process evaluation method. *Am. J. Public Health* 83:561–567, 1993.

Windsor, R., T. Baranowski, N. Clark, and G. Cutter. *Evaluation of Health Promotion,*

Health Education, and Disease Prevention Programs. Mountain View, CA: Mayfield, 1994.

Wonnacott, T. H., and R. J. Wonnacott. *Regression: A Second Course in Statistics.* Malabar, FL: Krieger Publishing Company, 1987.

Worthen, B. The unvarnished truth about logic-in-use and reconstructed logic in educational inquiry. *Eval. Pract.* 16:165–178, 1995.

Wulfert, E., and C. K. Wan. Condom use: a self-efficacy model. *Health Psychol.* 12: 346–353, 1993.

Index